Ebola Myths & Facts
FOR DUMMIES
A Wiley Brand

by Edward Chapnick, MD

Director, Division of Infectious Diseases
Vice Chair, Department of Medicine
Maimonides Medical Center, Brooklyn, N.Y.

Ebola Myths & Facts For Dummies®

Published by: **John Wiley & Sons, Inc.,** 111 River Street, Hoboken, NJ 07030-5774, www.wiley.com

Copyright © 2015 by John Wiley & Sons, Inc., Hoboken, New Jersey

Published simultaneously in Canada

For general information on our other products and services, please contact our Customer Care Department within the U.S. at 877-762-2974, outside the U.S. at 317-572-3993, or fax 317-572-4002. For technical support, please visit www.wiley.com/techsupport.

Wiley publishes in a variety of print and electronic formats and by print-on-demand. Some material included with standard print versions of this book may not be included in e-books or in print-on-demand. If this book refers to media such as a CD or DVD that is not included in the version you purchased, you may download this material at http://booksupport.wiley.com. For more information about Wiley products, visit www.wiley.com.

All photos printed courtesy of the Centers for Disease Control and Prevention's Public Health Image Library http://phil.cdc.gov/phil/home.asp.

Library of Congress Control Number: 2014957355

ISBN: 978-1-119-06622-4

ISBN 978-1-119-06622-4 (pbk); ISBN 978-1-119-06621-7 (ebk); ISBN 978-1-119-06626-2 (ebk)

Manufactured in the United States of America

10 9 8 7 6 5 4 3 2 1

Contents at a Glance

Table of Contents

Chapter 5: Receiving a Diagnosis and Undergoing Treatment........................55

Part III: Looking at Today and into the Future.... 69

Chapter 6: Eyeing the Geopolitical Outlook and Impact 71

Introduction

*E*bola.

It's on most people's minds to varying degrees. Some people watch the news coverage and wonder what it all means. You've probably seen the devastation in West Africa and wonder how it could have happened so fast and when it will end. You've seen cases come overseas into the United States, and you ask if the United States (and possibly Canada and Western Europe) is next for a big outbreak. Some people are seeing new policies at work and in public places as a result of a heightened public awareness. You may even be right in the thick of things, battling on the front lines to stop the current outbreak in West Africa from getting worse and doing what you can to help the people who need it most.

Once upon a time a public health emergency in West Africa may have felt far away, remote, and not applicable to you. But in today's global society — with technology and mass travel and family members and friends spread out in all directions — an emergency anywhere can feel like it's right in your own backyard.

Wherever you are, whatever you're doing, chances are good that Ebola has somehow impacted your life, even if it's just to prompt your curiosity to know more about this virus and outbreak — and maybe even public health in general.

This outbreak is a scary yet fascinating experience. The Ebola outbreak of 2014 is unprecedented, and the world is trying to figure out how to respond together. From providing care on the front lines to educating communities to examining world health policy, the outbreak is a complex issue to make sense of and do something about. Science, history, and politics have intersected, and it's everyone's job to discover as much as possible to help stop the crisis in West Africa, keep everyone safe and sound all across the world — at home and abroad — and move forward as a world united with a mission to prevent something like this outbreak in the future.

About This Book

People are trying to process what's happening, and what they can and should do about it. Reading *Ebola Myths & Facts For Dummies* is a good start. It contains no hype, no spin. It's just the facts, ma'am (or sir), and it's meant to give you a thorough, yet easy-to-understand guide.

It presents the basics (like how you can prevent yourself from getting Ebola), and also touches on some of the more layered issues, such as the ways different countries have responded to this outbreak. It does this all in plain English, sharing as much factual information as possible, rather than going on about my opinions or theories.

This book is a reference tool you can turn to in order to understand whatever particular aspect of Ebola you want. The beauty is that you don't have to read through the entire book cover to cover to get the information you want. You can simply open to the table of contents, find what you're looking for, and head directly to that section.

You can expect to find useful reference material such as:

✔ How this virus was discovered and how it led to this outbreak (refer to Chapter 2)

✔ How to know if someone has Ebola (head to Chapter 5)

✔ What to expect and how to prepare if you're a health worker heading into the affected areas (check out Chapter 7)

✔ A quick rundown of the most common myths busted (flip to Chapter 8)

Foolish Assumptions

In order to write something that was clear and helpful, I had to zero in on who I thought would read this book. So even though I never like to assume, I have to admit, I did make a few assumptions here in this book about you as my readers:

✔ You have heard or seen at least something about Ebola in the news or maybe from a friend or co-worker.

✔ You have come here to discover the facts on Ebola.

> ✔ You probably aren't in an affected area right now, but may be in the near future.
>
> ✔ You care about keeping yourself (and others) safe and healthy.
>
> ✔ You have a basic understanding of or experience with common illnesses like the flu and colds.

Icons Used in This Book

Look for those familiar *For Dummies* icons to offer visual clues about the kinds of material you're about to read.

 This icon points out some good advice relating to the subject matter you're reading about. Skimming these icons can give you some good tips to help you navigate the different steps in staying healthy (and helping others do the same)!

 The information that you're reading about and potentially sharing with others can be serious and impactful. I highlight important concepts and facts with this icon. Consider these the "extra-important" paragraphs you'll want to remember.

 This icon points out information that is meant to steer you away from harmful or dangerous situations. Be sure always to read these.

 The icon directs you to additional online information about Ebola. You can find it at www.dummies.com/extras/ebolamythsandfacts.

Beyond the Book

In addition to the content of this book, you can access some valuable related material online.

You can read a free Cheat Sheet at www.dummies.com/cheatsheet/ebolamythsandfacts that gives you all the information you want the most in a fast and easy way (like a list of Ebola symptoms and what to do if you think someone you know has it), without having to go through pages and pages of text. Remembering all the facts about Ebola can be difficult, so the cheat sheet is also a great tool to recollect what you read here.

You can also access some additional helpful bits of information at www.dummies.com/extras/ebolamythsandfacts. I cover some extra topics, such as common scenarios from which you can't contract Ebola and how to fight the stigma of Ebola.

Where to Go from Here

The book is about as modular as you can get with this topic. Each chapter contains a bunch of information and is self-contained, meaning that you don't have to read one chapter to understand what happens in the next. If there's something you saw on TV or you only care about how not to catch Ebola, use the table of contents as your guide and skip right to the appropriate chapter to read about it.

Chapter 1 is a great place to start to get your bearings in the book. Suppose you do want to read about the symptoms of Ebola and how to prevent getting it, you can head to Chapter 5. Start with Chapter 3 if you want all the details on the current situation in West Africa. If you're a healthcare worker who's heading to an affected area and need to cut right to the chase so you can prepare yourself, go to Chapter 7. And if you want to explore the science and evolution of Ebola, your starting point is Chapter 2.

The easiest way, though, to use the book is to start turning pages and read the content. And because I know that this topic is very important and concerning to many folks, don't be shy about making notes in the chapters, highlighting information, and putting flags on the pages so you can come back later.

Oh, and one more note: If you're reading this because you feel ill, put this book down and get thee to a doctor!

Part I
Getting Started with Ebola Myths & Facts

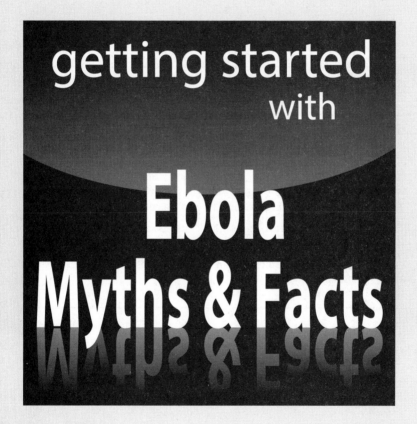

getting started
with

Ebola
Myths & Facts

Go to www.dummies.com/cheatsheet/ebolamythsandfacts for a cheat sheet chockfull of content about Ebola, including the common symptoms and modes of transmission.

In this part . . .

- ✔ Explore how Ebola was discovered and what scientists have been able to figure out about the virus.

- ✔ Chronicle the historical Ebola outbreaks since its discovery more than 35 years ago and identify the different countries of the world that have had confirmed cases and deaths.

- ✔ Uncover the parts of the world where Ebola affects people and what makes those people the most vulnerable.

- ✔ Examine the 2014 outbreak, including how it started and how it spread so quickly.

Chapter 1

The Lowdown on Ebola

*T*his chapter serves as your road map to everything Ebola related. Some of the details about Ebola can be a little confusing or upsetting, but I try to make it as easy as possible to understand what's happening.

Researchers and scientists are still discovering so much about Ebola (after all, the virus isn't even 50 years old), but I can promise you that I share with you what is known. Keep in mind that things are changing rapidly because of the current active outbreak. This chapter gives you the basics of Ebola and serves as your jumping-off point.

Answering the 5 Ws and 1 H About Ebola

You may have heard of the 5 *Ws* of journalism — the who, what, when, where, and why of the story. The *H* of how usually gets thrown in there, too. The concept is meant to make sure journalists get all the important stuff into a news piece without leaving their audience hanging. These sections answer these questions to make sure that you have all the basic information before diving into all of the many details about Ebola.

Grasping what Ebola is

Ebola is a virus that results in a hemorrhagic fever (which is called Ebola). People can give it to one another, but it isn't very easy to contract. However, if someone does get it, it can be very serious. If not treated, Ebola causes flulike symptoms at first, then more serious organ failure, which can result in death. Ebola is in the news right now because of a large outbreak in West Africa that has spread slightly onto other continents, including North America.

If you're interested in the full evolution and behavior of the virus, Chapter 2 has more about the history and science of Ebola.

Understanding who Ebola affects the most

Currently, Ebola affects West Africans in Guinea, Sierra Leone, and Liberia — and the healthcare workers taking care of them — the most. These folks are right in the line of Ebola fire every day. They get no break. No reprieve. They're watching their friends and family members die as they struggle to survive.

Westerners in West Africa who hold different beliefs and cultural traditions than the residents are coordinating and driving a good deal of the humanitarian efforts. It can make a tragic situation even tenser, because aid workers have to be careful not to ostracize community members, but rather care for and work with them.

Many West Africans don't even believe that Ebola is caused by a virus, but rather a curse or black magic. As a result, when they see doctors in full body protection trying to take them or their loved ones away, they're upset.

Adding to the distress is knowing that a great number of people who go into the treatment centers don't make it out alive, leading to a conclusion that the treatment centers are killing patients.

Eyeing where Ebola makes its mark

Although a few cases have sprung up outside of West Africa, by far, the only geographic area of major concern for Ebola right now is in Liberia, Sierra Leone, and Guinea, and their immediate neighbors. Chapter 2 takes a closer look at these countries to paint a clearer picture why Ebola has affected so many people there.

But the bigger takeaway here is the importance of a substantial healthcare system in each country, and the value of a worldwide network and plan for responding to health emergencies. This outbreak is happening specifically in these countries because of a lack of sufficient infrastructure to provide the response and education needed to stop it (such as doctors, nurses, and hospitals for treatment; mass media for public health messages; and highways and developed transportation to get help fast). None of the other countries in which Ebola has surfaced has suffered so deeply because they have the resources to combat it.

This time, Ebola has struck West Africa, but many other places could be next. So the point is that voters need to pressure their representatives and lawmakers to make sure funding and resources stay in place (or get added where needed) in the United States and Canada — or wherever you call home — to provide for the proper establishment and upkeep of vital infrastructure.

Knowing when Ebola became a concern

Since Ebola was first discovered in 1976, it has had 35 outbreaks. All of them have been small — mostly less than 50 deaths, and none more than 300. Starting in December of 2013, Guinea experienced an outbreak of an unknown virus that took 50 lives. By March of 2014, Guinea figured out that it was Ebola, and Liberia and Sierra Leone each reported a few cases as well.

Doctors Without Borders recognized the signs of a widespread epidemic in the making and sounded the alarm in April. The organization was concerned that cases were being diagnosed in three different countries at the same time. (That's how the organization knew that there was a big problem.) The current case count for this outbreak is closing in on 14,500 at time of publication.

For more on the timeline and how the World Health Organization (WHO) and the rest of the world reacted to this news and are planning for the future, turn to Chapter 6.

Comprehending why Ebola is a global concern

In West Africa, this outbreak is leaving thousands of families destroyed. Children have become orphans, and survivors are being cast out for fear that they will still spread the disease or are somehow cursed. The agriculture, trade, and tourism industries in these areas have totally disintegrated, and the situation is especially dire in the hot zone countries of Guinea, Liberia, and Sierra Leone — and even in the countries that border them, such as Ivory Coast and Mali. And the reach of this crisis is being felt around the world.

Nobody wants to go to these countries, and people in these countries are finding it difficult to get out, due to travel and border restrictions.

The longer that fear perpetuates and drives policies and protocols that prohibit vital industry, the deeper the world will feel the impact of this virus. When countries aren't generating revenue, they aren't spending it. And when they aren't growing crops, they aren't exporting them, let alone eating any crops. Food insecurity is a real threat as supply and demand drives prices for produce up 150 percent in some areas.

All three countries had been on the economic upswing, but each of them now stands to lose between 2 and 9 percent of their respective GDPs.

Recent estimates by the CDC say case numbers could hit 1 million, and the World Bank estimates that this could cost $32 billion over the next two years if Ebola keeps spreading across West African borders. You can read more about the global impact in Chapter 6.

Examining how Ebola is transmitted

Ebola is transmitted only through direct contact with infected body fluids, which means that the fluid has to touch your mucus membrane or non-intact skin. And that's it. That's the only way you can contract it. So in other words, you can't:

- ✔ Transmit the virus unless you have symptoms
- ✔ Catch Ebola just by being in the same room as a patient with Ebola (because the virus isn't airborne)

Ebola actually is quite difficult to contract when you compare it to something like the flu. So then why has Ebola spread like wildfire in West Africa?

Well, the rate at which the virus has spread during this outbreak is unprecedented, so it was extremely unexpected and caught a lot of the world health leaders off guard. Ebola was spreading in epidemic proportions before anyone could get ahead of it. Here are a couple of reasons why:

- ✔ Ebola hit large, highly populated urban areas versus the remote, far-flung villages it has historically appeared in.

- ✔ West African funeral rituals involve a lot of touching and washing of the body. Because a lot of fluids are involved when someone dies of Ebola, multiple people were (still are) coming into contact with infected fluids regularly.

- ✔ The borders are very porous in this part of West Africa, so it's typical for folks to come from miles around and from other countries to attend funerals, and then go back to their country and spread the virus unknowingly.

Chapter 4 discusses transmission in greater depth.

Noticing the Symptoms

The tricky thing about Ebola is that the early symptoms are very common and can easily be confused with symptoms of everything from influenza to malaria. Symptoms in the early stages of Ebola include fever, headache, muscle pain, weakness, which could describe how I felt the last time I was in bed sick.

After the disease progresses, symptoms do change a bit and move into diarrhea, vomiting, and unexplained bruising and bleeding. Chapter 5 spells out the common symptoms.

What you really need to know about recognizing Ebola is that it's less about taking the symptoms at face value or looking at them in a vacuum and more about identifying them and comparing them to your exposure history.

Most people (especially outside of West Africa) who exhibit these symptoms *don't* have Ebola. So if you're sitting on your couch in Fort Worth, Texas, or Fort Wayne, Indiana, or St. Paul, Minnesota, or St. Augustine, Florida, wondering if your fever is Ebola, I can pretty much tell you that it's not.

Arming Yourself: Prevention Is Key

Preventing the spread of Ebola is remarkably simple and similar to any other virus prevention, so long as you're not in a hot zone in West Africa. But even if you're in a hot zone, some detailed protocols and safety gear and equipment can protect you.

Everything goes back to these prevention steps:

- ✔ Wash your hands frequently with warm water and soap or use an alcohol-based hand sanitizer.

- ✔ Avoid contact with the blood and body fluids of any person, particularly someone who is sick.

- ✔ Don't handle items that may have come in contact with an infected person's blood or body fluids.

- ✔ Don't touch the body of someone who has died from Ebola.

- ✔ Don't touch bats and nonhuman primates (apes and monkeys) or their blood and fluids, and don't touch or eat raw meat prepared from these animals.

- ✔ Avoid facilities in West Africa where Ebola patients are being treated. The US Embassy or consulate is often able to provide advice on medical facilities.

- ✔ Seek medical care immediately if you develop fever, fatigue, headache, muscle pain, diarrhea, vomiting, stomach pain, or unexplained bruising or bleeding.

Refer to Chapter 4 for more detailed information about how you can keep yourself safe from Ebola. The good news: Many of these prevention methods also work against other more common viruses, such as the flu and colds.

Beyond making sure people take care of themselves on an individual level, there are special considerations for you if you're a healthcare worker out in the field. Additionally, citizens of all countries should take it upon themselves to make sure their nation and the global community is as healthy as possible.

What to do if you're a healthcare worker

Being a healthcare worker in an affected area means that your life (and others') depends on how well you adhere to personal protective equipment (PPE) protocols, environmental cleaning protocols, and safe handling and interaction protocols when in situations like a funeral. But this information about protection is just the tip of the iceberg. In fact, I have a whole chapter just for you, so head to Chapter 7.

What society can do

As a whole, the first thing society can do is not panic. People in the United States, Canada, and Western Europe aren't in danger. You can take a deep breath and stop feeding into unnecessary hype. From there, you can:

- ✔ Continue to educate yourself by consuming news through reputable sources, such as the WHO website (www.who.org), the CDC website (www.cdc.gov), and the National Institutes of Health website (www.nih.gov).

- ✔ Maintain good regular hygiene, paying special attention to washing your hands with soap and warm water.

- ✔ Support efforts and funding to expand services in West Africa. If Ebola is dealt with there, it won't find its way here.

- ✔ Vote for representatives that back sound public health policies.

- ✔ Get your flu shot. Flu season is here, and you don't need to crowd the hospitals with a bunch of people who have symptoms that also look like Ebola. You don't need to freak out (including yourself and your loved ones). Plus, keep hospital space open for those who really need it.

- ✔ If someone you know thinks that he has Ebola-like symptoms, you can help by separating him in a room and calling the health department for further instruction.

Testing for Ebola

Symptoms alone don't tell the story. The only way to know for sure if someone has Ebola is to test him for it. Several tests can detect both the virus itself and the antibodies that fight it. Testing must be done in a medical setting, because it involves blood draws and laboratory analysis.

It can take several days of symptoms before the test will show positive for Ebola because the virus initially lives in your organs. Then, after it progresses and grows enough, it enters the blood stream, which is when the testing can detect it. Chapter 5 has more information about the different ways to test for Ebola.

If you suspect someone has Ebola, the protocol is fairly simple: You isolate the person (you can just put him in a separate room) and then call the health department for guidance.

The CDC's guidance on suspected Ebola patients is to "identify, isolate, and inform." This means that the first course of action is to identify exposure history to find out if the patient has been to a country with an outbreak or has been otherwise exposed to a known Ebola patient. Then, healthcare workers must note the symptoms that someone is exhibiting to determine if they are indeed Ebola-like. The response and care protocols that follow depend on the assessment of both of those identification processes.

Three levels of response are used when addressing suspected or confirmed Ebola patients: isolation, quarantine, and monitoring.

- ✔ If the patient has an exposure history and symptoms that are consistent with Ebola, he is isolated.

- ✔ If the patient has an exposure history but no symptoms, he is either quarantined or monitored.

For more information, turn to Chapter 4.

Undergoing Treatment

Ebola has no cure. No drug can knock it out and no vaccine can prevent it. Patients have to rely on their own immune systems to attack it. This is even more of a problem for people who have compromised immune systems or who don't have access to proper medical care.

Treatment for Ebola comes down to the following:

- ✔ Replacing the large amounts of fluid lost by sweating, vomiting, and diarrhea with IV fluids

- ✔ Managing pain

- ✔ Watching for signs of and pre-empting organ failure

Chapter 5 examines the different treatment options in greater detail.

Making a Recovery

Recovering from Ebola can take awhile, but people can recover from it. Ebola isn't necessarily a death sentence — and less so if you're recovering from it in a country where the medical facilities aren't already totally taxed. It can take a few weeks to become symptom-free and test clear for it, but you may have something like muscle or joint pain or fatigue that lasts for several months or more.

So how do you beat it?

Well, scientists don't exactly know yet, but they have some ideas about what helps:

- ✔ **The patient's immune system:** If it's generally healthy, the chance of recovery is greater.

- ✔ **Early diagnosis and access to treatment:** Those individuals with exposure risk who are on top of it and get treated at the slightest symptom are the ones who have a better chance.

- ✔ **The mode of transmission matters:** Needlestick cases seem anecdotally to take longer to recover (or don't recover at all) versus those that contract it through human-to-human contact.

Looking at the Future of Ebola

The outbreak isn't under control yet. It has ebbed and flowed. Some weeks it seems to be slowing down, with some countries even being declared Ebola-free by officials, only to have another case surface. Progress is being made in small steps, but it's going to take quite some time still for healthcare workers to rein the outbreak in and halt it (in fact, the UN estimates the current outbreak won't be contained until mid 2015). The main thing is that they can't let up on the frontlines. And non-affected countries must keep the aid flowing into and the focus on West Africa. Head to Chapter 6 to read more about all the layers this outbreak impacts.

Eyeing West Africa: At most risk

Of all the people and entities that are affected and at risk, no one is more vulnerable than West Africa. Those countries are in the midst of a public health emergency, and it will be extremely difficult for them to recover, even after the outbreak is contained. All aspects of their society are impacted in these ways:

- ✔ They're facing a food crisis because the Ebola outbreak has been happening throughout their harvest time. Labor forces are being lost to sickness, and even people who are still well enough to work often can't access farms due to border regulations.

✔ Airline restrictions have made travel (including that for trade) nearly impossible, which means that tourism has been eliminated almost entirely and foreign citizens are being pulled out by their countries.

✔ Even just daily life is a struggle at the moment. Children have been orphaned, entire families have been wiped out, and survivors are being ostracized and demonized.

Providing help

In this type of situation, all hands on deck are needed. Although controversy surrounds how world health leaders and other powers handled the initial outbreak, funding and efforts are now well underway. Without the help of nations from around the globe, West Africa won't be able to stop the outbreak. Millions of dollars are being contributed as well as many tons of supplies. Volunteers, such as healthcare professionals, health education specialists, case workers, and logistics managers, are on the frontlines providing life-saving care, education, and assistance while people in the United States and Canada can participate by donating and sharing the right information.

So what kinds of tasks and projects are volunteers doing in West Africa, besides providing direct medical care? Some of the work includes

✔ Receiving and sorting supplies

✔ Mapping affected areas and tracking cases

✔ Planning and building new mobile clinics and labs

✔ Working with communities to educate residents in effective and innovative ways about Ebola prevention and response

✔ Providing social services to survivors, including orphaned children

✔ Tracking contacts of confirmed Ebola patients

✔ Compiling data and research

If you want to know how you can help, check out Chapter 9 that lists ten organizations that are contributing to the efforts.

Chapter 2

Examining the Science and History of Ebola

*P*eople colloquially use the word *Ebola* as an all-encompassing word actually to describe two different things:

✔ **A virus (its full name *Ebolavirus*):** This virus seems to be related to the viruses that cause measles and mumps. Scientists are still learning about this virus, its behavior, where it comes from, and how to develop a vaccine for it.

✔ **The disease that results from the virus (full name *Ebola hemorrhagic fever*):** Being a *hemorrhagic fever virus* means that it causes fluid to leak from blood vessels, resulting in a dangerously low drop in blood pressure.

No matter which you mean, Ebola is one of the world's deadliest viruses and diseases. It's a merciless killer with a death rate of up to 90 percent.

The only possible good thing about Ebola is that although it's extremely infectious, it's not very contagious. This chapter takes you through the basic science and history of Ebola so that you can get to know a little more about it.

Knowing What a Virus Is

A *virus* is a microscopic organism that can reproduce without any sort of host and then infiltrate all types of organisms (animals, plants, bacteria, and fungi) — and viruses are everywhere. There are millions of viruses all over the world, and they exist in pretty much every ecosystem on earth.

Although most people think of viruses as bad, some viruses are actually good. Many of them perform helpful tasks. For example, viruses are key in the process of decomposition, particularly in the ocean. As viruses decompose other organisms, they generate and release carbon dioxide, which then feeds the marine plant life.

Viruses were first identified in the 19th century and were initially grouped separately from other microorganisms based on the fact that they were small enough to pass through filters that bacteria couldn't.

Viruses spread in many ways:

- ✓ Between plants by insects that feed on sap
- ✓ By blood-sucking insects (otherwise known as *vectors*)
- ✓ Through coughing and sneezing
- ✓ Through feces
- ✓ Through semen and vaginal fluid
- ✓ Through exposure to infected blood and other body fluids

Ebola spreads through infected blood and other body fluids (including feces, semen, and vaginal fluid); refer to Chapter 4 for more on Ebola transmission.

Infections prompt a person's immune system to fight and eliminate the infecting virus (or other germ). *Antibodies* are one part of the immune system, and they're very specific — sort of like a lock and key. If you've been infected with a certain germ, the antibodies produced protect you from that specific organism and no others. This is the basis for immunization, which utilizes specific components of the *pathogen,* or a live inactivated version of the germ, to produce an antibody response. For Ebola, the antibodies to each specific species are different. Although scientists have been researching Ebola immunizations for several years, none have yet to be approved. The good news is that several immunizations in development show promise.

Antibiotics have no effect on viruses, so they clearly aren't a viable treatment for people with Ebola. Chapter 5 discusses treatment options for patients infected with Ebola.

Discovering Ebola

In 1976, a blood sample from a Belgian nun who died in Zaire (now known as the Democratic Republic of the Congo) was sent to a lab in Belgium. At first, doctors thought that she had yellow fever, but after further analysis, the scientists realized that it was something different and sent the sample to the CDC, which then confirmed it was an unknown virus — a virus that would come to be known as Ebola.

That outbreak had 318 reported cases and 280 deaths. A separate outbreak also occurred in Sudan (now South Sudan) and resulted in 284 cases and 151 deaths.

Since the initial discovery, researchers have uncovered some information about Ebola, even though they have much to learn. These sections identify the different species that researchers have discovered and the different Ebola outbreaks in the past 40 years.

Identifying the five species of Ebola

Ebolavirus (EBOV) is one of three known viruses within the family *Filoviridae*. EBOV has five different species, and four of the five cause a severe and often fatal hemorrhagic fever in humans and other mammals, known as Ebola virus disease (EVD).

The five different species/strains of the Ebola virus are

- ✔ Zaire (the 2014 outbreak is this strain)
- ✔ Bundibugyo
- ✔ Sudan
- ✔ Reston
- ✔ Tai Forest

The first three have been associated with large outbreaks in Africa. The Zaire and Sudan strains are the most common and most deadly for humans. The Bundibugyo and Tai Forest strains have been seen only a few times. The identification of the Reston subtype of Ebola is also of interest. Scientists identified it in dying monkeys imported to a research facility from the Philippines. Although some exposed humans were found to have antibodies, indicating that they had become infected, none became sick.

Ebola also has a deadly distant cousin. Go to www.dummies.com/extras/ebolamythsandfacts for more information about the Marburg virus.

Eyeing the outbreaks

Since its discovery, more than 35 outbreaks of Ebola (including the 2014 one) have been documented. The current 2104 outbreak is the largest in history. Table 2-1 lists the full history of Ebola outbreaks.

Table 2-1	The History of Ebola Outbreaks	
Year	*Country*	*Deaths*
1976	Zaire	280
1976	Sudan	151
1976	England	0
1977	Zaire	1
1979	Sudan	22
1989	United States	0
1990	United States	0
1989–1990	Philippines	0
1992	Italy	0
1994	Gabon	31
1994	Ivory Coast	0
1995	Democratic Republic of the Congo (DRC)	250
1996 (January to April)	Gabon	21
1996 - 1997 (July to January)	Gabon	45
1996	South Africa	1
1996	United States	0
1996	Philippines	0

Year	Country	Deaths
1996	Russia	1
2000–2001	Uganda	224
2001–2002 (October to March)	Gabon	53
2001–2002 (October to March)	DRC	43
2002–2003 (December to April)	DRC	128
2003	DRC	29
2004	Sudan	1
2004	Russia	1
2007	DRC	187
2007–2008 (December to January)	Uganda	37
2008	Philippines	0
2008–2009 (December to February)	DRC	15
2011	Uganda	1
2012	Uganda	4
2012	DRC	13
2012–2013 (November to January)	Uganda	3
March 2014 to present	Multiple countries	(ongoing; see Chapter 3)
August 2014 to present	DRC	(ongoing; see Chapter 3)

Understanding How Ebola Works

Ebola is a *zoonotic* disease, which means that it occurs naturally in animals but that it can be transmitted to humans. Researchers aren't sure yet which animal(s) are the hosts, but the frontrunner is the fruit bat. One of the biggest reasons that determining the host has been so difficult is that Ebola outbreaks *ebb and flow,* suggesting a rare species might be the host. Chapter 4 provides more information about transmission.

Some virus particles have a spherical shape, but the Ebola's particles are filament-like in structure, which gives them more surface area to potentially attack a greater number of cells. *Filo* is Latin for *filament,* which describes the shape of the virus. Figure 2-1 shows what the Ebola virus looks like.

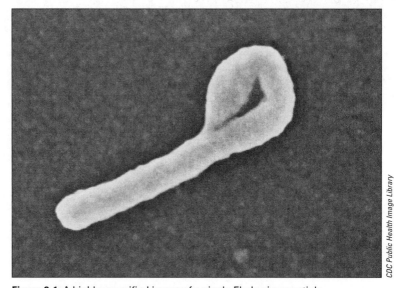

CDC Public Health Image Library

Figure 2-1: A highly magnified image of a single Ebola virus particle.

All viruses have *attachment proteins,* also referred to as *glycoproteins.* Part of what makes Ebola so infectious is that its long, filament-shaped virus particle is completely covered by these glycoproteins. The glycoproteins find a healthy cell, attach to it (that connection point is called a *receptor site*), and then the Ebola virus can enter the cell and the immune system, replicating itself as it goes.

Just like other viruses, after Ebola infects a person's cells, it triggers the release of a bunch of different types of chemicals within the person's body. These chemicals and cells are actually the immune response to the infection. If this response isn't properly modulated, it can cause serious disease or death from infection. *Sepsis* refers to the systemic inflammatory (or immune) response to infection, which can be fatal.

In addition to the virus having a ton of glycoproteins, it's also fairly impartial and will infect a wide range of cell types in the human body. Early on in the disease, Ebola typically invades a certain type of white blood cells associated with the immune system called *T cells* (short for *t lymphocyte*). After that early infection, it travels to the lymph nodes, spleen, and liver through the blood.

The time it takes for a person to show symptoms after the Ebola virus has initially attacked her system can be anywhere from 2 to 21 days, which is called the *incubation period.* On average, people start showing symptoms within eight to ten days. Many factors influence how quickly symptoms progress and the immune system deteriorates, so the earlier a person identifies her symptoms and gets treated, the better her chances of recovery are. Refer to Chapter 5 for more information.

Explaining the Biosafety Level of Ebola

All disease-causing organisms are classified in one of four levels of *biological safety levels.* The Centers for Disease Control and Prevention (CDC) developed and administer the levels to make sure that scientists who are studying these organisms know how dangerous they are and how to protect themselves against infection. Each level has protocols for categorizing and safely handling and storing the organisms. Level 1 (BSL-1) indicates the most innocuous and benign of organisms. Level 4 is the most dangerous. Ebola is at BSL-4.

Currently, seven operational labs in the United States are designated BSL-4 and can therefore do Ebola research. They are as follows:

- ✔ CDC in Atlanta, Georgia (two labs are located there)

- ✔ Center for Biodefense and Emerging Infectious Diseases (University of Texas Medical Branch) in Galveston, Texas

- ✔ Southwest Foundation for Biomedical Research in San Antonio, Texas

- ✔ US Army Medical Research Institute for Infectious Diseases (Department of Defense) in Frederick, Maryland

- ✔ Rocky Mountain Laboratories Integrated Research Facility (National Institute of Allergy and Infectious Diseases) in Hamilton, Montana

Six more are under construction or planned. They include

- ✔ Integrated Research Facility (National Institute of Allergy and Infectious Diseases) in Fort Detrick, Maryland

- ✔ Galveston National Laboratory (University of Texas Medical Branch) in Galveston, Texas

- ✔ National Biodefense Analysis and Countermeasures Center (Department of Homeland Security) in Frederick, Maryland

- ✔ National Bio- and Agro-Defense Facility (Department of Homeland Security) in Manhattan, Kansas

- ✔ National Biocontainment Laboratory (Boston University) in Boston, Massachusetts

- ✔ Virginia Division of Consolidated Laboratory Services (Department of General Services of the Commonwealth of Virginia) in Richmond, Virginia

Figure 2-2 gives you an idea of just how much gear scientists need to wear when studying the world's most dangerous viruses.

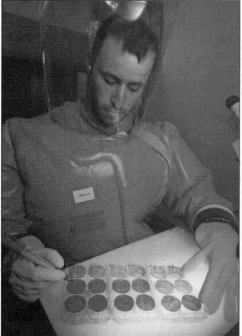

CDC Public Health Image Library

Figure 2-2: A microbiologist wears full protective gear while working in the CDC BSL-4 lab.

Chapter 3

Taking a Closer Look at the 2014 Outbreak

. . . .

In This Chapter

▶ Understanding how the 2014 outbreak started and is spreading specifically in West Africa

▶ Considering the other parts of the world that have seen Ebola

▶ Identifying the public health entities responding to the outbreak

▶ Deciding whether you need to panic or not

. . . .

*T*he 2014 Ebola outbreak is the largest and most complex in history. Although it mostly remains in West Africa, the outbreak has garnered international attention from all corners of the globe, prompting concern and even hysteria. Countries all over the world have responded to the needs in West Africa and continue to prepare their own citizens for prevention and treatment, should it reach their borders. Countries that have encountered isolated cases have instituted measures, such as travel bans, robust screenings at hospitals and airports, and mandatory quarantines. The unfortunate part is that the governments (particularly in the United States) don't seem to be investing the same energy into public education efforts. Hence, even though the extensive media coverage of Ebola is at a fever pitch, people aren't quite getting the full picture.

This chapter breaks down exactly how this recent outbreak started, what the current state of affairs is, and how concerned you should be about your own safety.

Eyeing Ground Zero: West Africa

The Ebola outbreak of 2014 is currently a full-blown health crisis in West Africa. Although the numbers of those affected are fluid and constantly changing, the World Health Organization, also known as WHO (read more about it in the section "Managing and Responding to the Current Outbreak" later in this chapter) estimates that the average Ebola death rate is approximately 50 percent. At the time of publication, more than 15,000 cases and 5,400 deaths had been reported in West Africa due to Ebola, which makes the overall death rate around 37 percent; however, that number increases when you look at individual countries.

During an outbreak, fatality rates are almost always underestimated. Here are some reasons why:

- ✔ **The case count includes individuals who are very early on in the illness, but who will eventually die.** They may die for any number of reasons, such as not getting treatment early enough or not having a strong enough immune system to begin with (more on what it takes to recover from Ebola in Chapter 5). Therefore, the number of deaths will continue to increase even after the last new case has occurred.

  For example, say that at a given point in time, there are 100,000 cases and 50,000 deaths, which seems like an overall 5 percent death rate. However, of the 100,000 cases, say that 10,000 are currently ill, and 7,000 of these will eventually die. (This is just an example; the number here will never be zero.) In this case, the actual mortality rate will be 57 percent, not what appears to be 50 percent.

- ✔ **In some areas, health officials don't report deaths accurately or on time because the medical centers are so overwhelmed.** Liberia and Sierra Leone's healthcare systems were essentially non-existent even before Ebola struck due to the civil wars that decimated their infrastructures. Guinea's system was a little better off to begin with (the country has been actively reorganizing and investing in its healthcare infrastructure since 1987), but now that the outbreak is in full swing, all three countries' systems are inundated with patients, even with the international relief efforts.

- ✔ **Some deaths that happen in the villages aren't reported at all because some local residents don't trust the westernized way of handling the outbreak.** I discuss more about why they mistrust in Chapter 4.

These sections examine the countries in West Africa that faced Ebola outbreaks in 2014 and some explanations as to why this area of the world is more susceptible to Ebola.

Identifying the affected countries

Ebola has hit three of the countries in West Africa the hardest. Some reports suggest that the increase of deforestation in West Africa for mining purposes and a longer and drier season than usual has pushed fruit bats closer to human habitats, thereby increasing the amount of exposure villagers have to the virus hosts. Chapter 2 explains in greater depth the role that bats play in the Ebola outbreak.

Figure 3-1 shows a map of the Western African countries most affected. The 2014 Ebola outbreak actually began in Guinea in December 2013 and then spread to Sierra Leone and Liberia. Nigeria and Senegal had small outbreaks, but both of those countries have been cleared of Ebola as of October 2014.

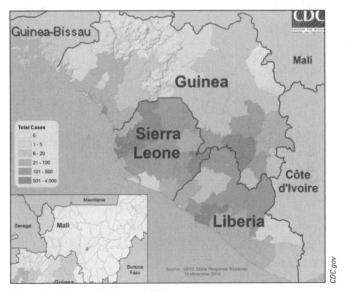

Figure 3-1: A map of Western Africa.

Guinea

Guinea, formerly known as French Guinea and sometimes referred to as Guinea-Conakry, is a country of approximately 10.5 million people located due north of Sierra Leone and Liberia. The current outbreak started with a 2-year-old in Guinea, referred to as *Patient 0* in the media. Nobody knows for sure how he initially contracted Ebola, but one theory is that his family hunted fruit bats, which is very common in that country and region. Shortly after his death, his mother, sister, and grandmother also died from Ebola. People from around the area attending the funerals and burial rituals for the family contracted the virus unknowingly and brought it with them when they went back over the borders to go home.

Local health authorities estimate that 60 percent of all cases in Guinea are linked to funerals and burials of those who have died from Ebola. See Chapter 4 for more information on how local burial rituals have spread the virus. At publication time, the current case count in Guinea is 1,760, with 1,054 deaths, which is a death rate of about 60 percent.

Liberia

Surrounded on three sides by Sierra Leone, Guinea, and Ivory Coast, Liberia has been mentioned in most of the news concerning the present outbreak. Liberia is the only country in Africa founded by US colonization when many freed slaves settled there in 1820. During the past 35 years, the country has faced economic and political upheaval.

Liberia's Ebola outbreak began in March, probably due to travel from Guinea. For much of the outbreak, Liberia was the country whose caseload of infected patients grew the fastest and most exponentially. In fact, the crisis level is the highest there out of any of the affected countries, mainly because of the number of cases in the densely populated capital of Monrovia and an intense mistrust of government, healthcare workers, and community activist directives — particularly in the slum of West Point. Additionally, the lack of beds and overall poor health system exacerbates the situation.

The good news is that the case rate in Liberia appears to be decreasing. At time of publication, 6,919 cases have been reported with 2,766 deaths. However because the situation is so dire, the true death toll may never be known, mostly due to improper reporting and disposal of bodies.

Sierra Leone

Sierra Leone is on the west coast of Africa and borders Guinea and Liberia. A civil war plagued the country from 1991 to 2002, forcing two million refugees across the borders.

The first confirmed case of Ebola in Sierra Leone during the 2014 outbreak was a woman admitted to a hospital for miscarriage in May. She recovered from the virus, and local community health workers determined that she likely had contracted it from a healer who lived and worked in her village. Hundreds of people who were sick with Ebola had visited the healer, who then contracted the virus and spread it to others.

Additionally, the healer's funeral drew hundreds of mourners. Because of the attendees' observation of and participation in traditional funeral rituals, they also contracted the virus. In fact, up to 365 deaths may be attributed to that one funeral. At time of publication, 4,862 cases of Ebola have been reported in Sierra Leone with 1,130 deaths.

Nigeria and Senegal

Two countries, Nigeria and Senegal, had isolated illnesses that were swiftly dealt with, which prevented Ebola from becoming widespread. Senegal shares borders with Mali and Guinea, whereas Nigeria is the most populous country in Africa.

A small outbreak began in Nigeria in July when an infected traveler from Liberia — who lied about his health status and history — arrived at a Nigerian airport. At the end of the country's outbreak (declared in October by WHO), Nigeria had had only 20 reported cases and eight deaths. This small caseload (relative to outbreaks in Sierra Leone, Guinea, and Liberia) is due to the country's fast and furious response. Health officials did what they were supposed to, in terms of quickly identifying and isolating patients, tracing, and monitoring their contacts, and those actions worked in preventing Ebola from spreading. (I discuss the importance of these actions in Chapters 5 and 7.)

Senegal was even more effective in preventing the spread of Ebola than Nigeria. In August, a traveler who had contact with an Ebola patient arrived from Guinea. The government's swift and proper response enabled the patient to recover and prevented Ebola from spreading to anyone else.

Granted independence from France in 1960, the citizens of Senegal speak French and are primarily Muslim. The country has strong relations with the West, especially France and the United States. As well, it's been a member of the UN Security Council and UN Commission on Human Rights.

Mali

Mali is one of the poorest countries in the world, but the United States has an ever-strengthening relationship with the country due to Mali's evolving pro-Western stance and desire to resolve conflict in the area (such as in Liberia and Sierra Leone).

On October 23, a 2-year-old in Mali who had traveled through Guinea tested positive for Ebola and became that country's first case. She died the next day, but because of Mali's swift and proper response, the Ebola virus didn't spread, and Mali was nearly declared Ebola-free until another case appeared on November 10 — this time a nurse in a private clinic. Doctors determined through genetic analysis and contact tracing that the two cases weren't linked; however, the second case also came from Guinea, when a man with Ebola sought treatment at the same hospital at which the nurse worked.

Additionally, because the man was a *grand imam* (a religious figure in the Islam faith), many people attended his funeral, generating a fear that this round of the outbreak could be substantially larger than the first. This turned out to be true, and at time of publication, Mali has had six Ebola cases and all patients have died.

As a result, Mali health officials have intensified its contact tracing and monitoring and currently have about 95 percent of the 327 identified contacts under daily monitoring for symptoms.

Discovering why Ebola has spread so far and fast in West Africa

The questions of why and how Ebola has spread so far and so fast in West Africa during 2014 are the subjects of much debate and analysis. Among some of the answers are the following:

- **Poor infrastructure:** This part of the world doesn't have a well-developed infrastructure. Things such as running water, sanitation, and healthcare systems are severely lacking. For example, the number of physicians in the affected countries was one to four per 100,000 people before the onset of the Ebola outbreak, which made it impossible for doctors to get control of the outbreak, even from the beginning.

- **Inexperience:** Although some countries (like Nigeria) have had experience with responding to large epidemics, many other countries (like Liberia) haven't had experience.

- **Delayed response:** The global healthcare leaders and policy makers didn't agree quickly enough with Doctors Without Borders that the epidemic would or could be as big as it is, and therefore, response was delayed. Chapter 6 discusses this point in more detail.

✔ **Urban areas affected:** In addition to remote, low-density villages, the outbreak has hit high-density urban areas. This is different from many of the outbreaks in the past. (I review the Ebola outbreak history in Chapter 2.) Urban areas contain more people that live closer together, are more mobile, and interact with each other at a higher frequency than remote villages do, enabling the virus to spread even faster.

✔ **Cultural divide:** Local residents and westerners typically have significantly different cultural values. Many locals' beliefs (especially concerning sickness and death) cause them to not abide by directives given by health officials. Many locals believe that the cause of this sickness and death isn't a virus that can be treated or prevented, but rather black magic. Many locals who were ill or who had sick family members rather would seek the help of a local healer or witch doctor than a western physician. Treatment by these healers proves to be fatal in most cases, because Ebola patients require intensive medical care to have a reasonable chance at survival.

Western physicians frighten many locals who view the physicians as taking away their loved ones where their loved ones often end up dying. (If they do attempt to receive medical help, Ebola patients often wait too long to seek it, severely limiting their chances for survival.) Additionally, the care provided in many of the local understaffed, poorly equipped, and overcrowded hospitals isn't adequate to treat these seriously ill people. Locals then make the faulty (but understandable) deduction that the doctors are killing their people.

Furthermore, the western approach of isolating Ebola patients to treat them harshly conflicts with many West African beliefs surrounding illness and death, which involves extensive contact with the sick and dying. Refer to Chapter 4 for more information about this.

Additionally, people in these areas are naturally skeptical of government and authorities, given their past with intense civil war and corruption, and won't even let western health officials be in their homes or villages.

✔ **Hopelessness:** With such a high fatality rate, some people don't think there's any point in going to a hospital, because they think death is inevitable.

✔ **Fear of hospital germs:** The loved ones of sick people don't want to take them to the hospital for fear that they will contract Ebola from the hospital.

Elsewhere in Africa: The Democratic Republic of the Congo

The Democratic Republic of Congo (DRC) in Central Africa also experienced an unrelated, independent (as proven by genetic analysis) Ebola outbreak in 2014.

It started in August with a woman who butchered a bush animal that most likely had the virus. She eventually died, and the virus then spread to the healthcare workers who performed local death rituals for her. Now more than 67 Ebola cases have been reported with 49 related deaths for an overall death rate of 74 percent. The WHO officially declared the DRC Ebola-free on November 21, 2014.

Focusing on the United States and Western Europe

Although the 2014 Ebola outbreak continues to hit West Africa the hardest, countries outside of that region have also seen minor caseloads. Read on for more about them.

United States

Although the media has sensationalized Ebola in the United States, only ten cases of Ebola have been treated in the United States in 2014. The first one diagnosed in September was a Liberian national who had travelled from West Africa to Dallas, Texas. His death is the subject of controversy and lawsuits because he originally went to the hospital complaining of symptoms, but the hospital staff sent him home. He returned three days later with progression of symptoms, tested positive for Ebola, and then died ten days later.

Eight of the other nine survived. The one who died was already very ill when he arrived in the United States. Some of them contracted and/or were diagnosed with the virus in the United States, whereas others contracted the virus in West Africa and evacuated to the United States for treatment. You can see the breakdown in Table 3-1.

Table 3-1	Ebola Cases in the United States during the 2014 Outbreak	
Cases Diagnosed in the United States	***Cases Evacuated to the United States***
Liberian national visitor to Dallas died in October after being treated for a week.	Doctor infected in Liberia, flown to Atlanta, and recovered in August with experimental drug after almost three weeks. Donated blood for other Ebola patients to use through transfusion.
Nurse infected while caring for Liberian national in Dallas in October and recovered after two weeks.	Missionary infected in Liberia, flown to Emory University in Atlanta, treated with experimental medication, and recovered in August after two weeks.
Nurse, also infected while caring for Liberian national in Dallas in October, called CDC to report fever, but was cleared to fly. She tested positive two days later, was treated, and recovered after a week and a half.	Missionary and also a doctor infected in Liberia, flown to Nebraska in September, treated with experimental medication and transfusion from recovered doctor's donation, and recovered.
Doctor infected while in West Africa with Doctors Without Borders, called ahead of his arrival back to the United States to warn he may be a high-risk case. His treatment in New York included an experimental medication and he recovered after two weeks.	Unidentified WHO doctor infected in Sierra Leone in September, flown to Emory, and recovered in October after a week.
	NBC cameraman infected in Liberia, flown to Nebraska in October, and recovered in two weeks.
	Doctor infected in Sierra Leone, flown to Nebraska in November, and died two days later.

All of the cases of Ebola in the United States originated in the affected area of West Africa. No one in the general population in the United States has contracted Ebola (even significant others living with quarantined individuals), due to several different factors:

✔ The United States has the capacity to handle the few cases that arrive here because the country isn't in the middle of a large outbreak.

✔ The United States has a well-developed healthcare system that already has facilities and trained professionals in place.

✔ The general public isn't exposed regularly to infected body fluids, which is how the virus is transmitted (visit Chapter 4 to read more about modes of transmission).

Spain

In August, Spain evacuated one of its citizens who was volunteering in Liberia and contracted the virus. He died a week later. Again in September, the country evacuated another infected Spaniard who was a missionary doing work in Sierra Leone. He died within a few days, and one of his healthcare workers also contracted the virus. She was treated in isolation and recovered a month later. At the time of publication, no other cases have been reported in Spain.

Other European countries

Norway, France, the United Kingdom, and Germany have also seen a small handful of cases. The European Union is dealing with the cases and public health in general similarly to the United States by performing extensive travel screening at the airports (which happens more frequently, given the greater number of flights that come from West Africa into Europe versus the United States), isolating anyone who is symptomatic and following up with concurrent contact tracing, and having well-stocked hospitals and trained staff to care for patients.

Ebola and man's best friend

After the healthcare worker in Spain was diagnosed with Ebola, the tracing efforts started and Spanish authorities focused on her pet dog, Excalibur. Despite international protests and local animal activists trying to physically prevent it, authorities euthanized him for fear that he was a reservoir host of the virus.

Euthanizing Excalibur is particularly sad, given that Bentley, the dog of one of the Dallas nurses who contracted Ebola, was quarantined and did well just a week later. Some evidence suggests that dogs may acquire Ebola, because they have been demonstrated to develop antibodies to the virus. However, no evidence shows that they either get sick from it or are able to transmit the virus.

Several European airlines have modified or suspended flights to West Africa, including Air France, British Airways, and Brussels Airlines.

Managing and Responding to the Current Outbreak

Many agencies and entities have had to work together to respond to a global epidemic. Without effective collaboration, sharing of resources, and involvement from all regions, a health crisis like the Ebola outbreak of 2014 won't end. These sections explain who (and what) is responsible for coordinating these massive efforts.

World Health Organization (WHO)

The World Health Organization (WHO) is the big boss when it comes to any sort of global healthcare concern.

The WHO's website (www.who.int/csr/disease/ebola/en/) explains the group's mission: "It is the directing and coordinating authority for health within the United Nations system. It is responsible for providing leadership on global health matters, shaping the health research agenda, setting norms and standards, articulating evidence-based policy options, providing technical support to countries and monitoring and assessing health trends." You can find lot more other helpful information at this site.

During this current outbreak, WHO has suffered some criticism (which I discuss more about in Chapter 6), but the organization is still considered the coordinating entity, working with various leaders, governments, and private agencies to produce a response that will be effective.

United Nations (UN)

The United Nations (UN) is an intergovernmental organization that's been in existence since 1945 with the mission of promoting international peace and security. It was founded after WWII to prevent another similar war from happening.

To address the current Ebola outbreak, the UN has formed the UN Mission for Ebola Emergency Response (UNMEER), which focuses mostly on helping with infrastructure needs, such as providing air assets, vehicles, and telecommunications. Refer to Chapter 6 for more information. You can also visit www.un.org/ebolaresponse/ - &panel1-1 for more specifics.

Centers for Disease Control and Prevention (CDC)

The Centers for Disease Control and Prevention (CDC) is the US government's major public health agency. It has a pretty large authority, but tends to defer to state and local health officials. During this outbreak response, the CDC has provided information and resources, such as logistics, staffing, analytics, communications, and management.

It, too, has been criticized for various missteps, especially early on, but it presses on and is working on new initiatives to battle this outbreak. Head to Chapter 6 for additional information about how the CDC has helped. You can also go to www.cdc.gov/vhf/ebola/ for more information.

State and local government/ health officials

State and local health officials are quite often the frontline first responders tasked with implementing the CDC's directives. They're the ones interfacing most directly with the public and potential and actual patients and healthcare workers.

In this current outbreak, they train healthcare facilities and their employees as well as law enforcement officers, and they also manage the laboratories that test for the virus. They communicate with and educate the public about Ebola. What's tricky about the state level is that the level of authority, care, and resources can vary from state to state.

For example, Governors Andrew Cuomo of New York and Chris Christie of New Jersey imposed a quarantine of Kaci Hickox, a nurse returning from West Africa, on October 24. (Refer to Chapter 4 for more specifics about these quarantines.) Fortunately, countries outside of the affected area haven't run into too many problems with consistency and organization because there haven't been many cases beyond Liberia, Guinea, and Sierra Leone.

Walking the Line between Valid Concern and Hysteria

The Ebola virus is spreading quickly in West Africa, and people are dying. The outbreak is definitely an emergency and warrants the serious response that it's getting. However, for the most part, people in the United States and Canada (and Western Europe) aren't at risk because of the modern infrastructure that provides things like running water, soap, and a well-established healthcare system. (I discuss the ins and outs of how Ebola is transmitted in Chapter 4.)

"But still," you may ask yourself, "isn't it *possible* that it could happen here, too, if we're not careful?" And "what about if it mutates?" Honestly, a virus has never mutated in a way that resulted in a change in the mode of transmission, so it's very unlikely that Americans and Canadians (and Western Europeans) are in danger. So why is everyone so panicked? Well, read on as I outline a few of the contributing factors to the current hysteria.

Common symptoms

The early symptoms of Ebola during the 2014 outbreak (and all other past Ebola outbreaks) are so commonplace that a person easily can get excited over what's ultimately just a cold or the flu. The common symptoms include coughing, sneezing, and feeling achy. Given that cold and flu season is in full swing as of this book's publication, many people currently have these symptoms, so it just adds to the public concern.

I discuss in more detail the symptoms of Ebola in Chapter 5, including the late-stage symptoms, which is what really sets Ebola apart from other illnesses.

Novelty

A major reason for the massive amounts of news coverage and individual worry in the United States and other western countries is that the general public doesn't know much about Ebola. People tend to fear what they don't understand. Although the flu is much more rampant than Ebola and kills thousands every year (due in part to the fact that only about 40 percent of Americans, 33 percent or less of Canadians, and as little as 2 percent of people in different EU countries actually get a flu shot every year), the flu doesn't receive the same coverage or response because people have gotten so desensitized to it.

Flu is more of a concern than Ebola, but it's old news and not as emotionally charged for people. Flu just doesn't *feel* like an emergency or crisis to most people because they've lived with it for so long. Society in general seems to have the attitude of, "sure, flu kills old people and babies sometimes, but it could never kill *me*." Nothing to see here and nothing to fear.

Media

The media is one of, if not *the*, biggest drivers behind the current frenzy. Although news coverage is important and informative, most of the news industry is a business in the end. As such, the great majority of news outlets operate with profits in mind, which means that they broadcast whatever will yield the highest ratings or largest reader/listenership. It also means that the media has a tendency to sensationalize or overhype stories in order to draw the audience in with drama.

When you read about something in the papers one day, then hear about it on the radio on the way to work, and *then* see the same thing on the news, it really grabs your attention, leading you (typically) to make the assessment that it must be important. But when that 24-7 news cycle continues reporting on the same issue for days, weeks, or months on end, you can shift from simply being concerned and interested to being paranoid and irrational.

Stories about Ebola are everywhere you turn, giving the impression that the United States is facing a major crisis — which is only partly true. The real crisis is in West Africa, and it definitely warrants the coverage. However, the coverage about the United States has been a bit overblown and contributes to public hysteria. You can help yourself avoid getting swept up in it by being a conscious news consumer and even doing your own research (like reading this book).

Travel

Airlines and other travel-based industries have enacted various protocols to prevent the current Ebola outbreak from spreading. As a result, when people travel, they have encountered these new policies. You see signage and witness procedures, which brings the Ebola outbreak even closer to home. You may even see someone get denied boarding or tended to in the middle of a flight. Not to mention, just being in a large public place like an airport exposes you to a lot of different people in various states of health and from various parts of the world.

Although the only part of the world that you need to be concerned about in regards to the current Ebola outbreak is West Africa, the heightened global concern tends to cause people to generalize and be suspicious of anyone coughing, sneezing, or feeling feverish while traveling.

Part II
Keeping Yourself Safe and Healthy

What you can do here to stop the epidemic

Sometimes, you can feel powerless to do anything to help the people who need it most because you are so far away. But there are things you can do:

- Use your votes to support candidates who back improvements in the public health system and not measures fueled by hysteria over science.
- Demand that Congress approves funding to help fight Ebola.
- Donate to organizations that are fighting Ebola in West Africa.
- Educate yourself on the facts so that you don't contribute to hysteria.
- Get a flu shot so that you don't overwhelm the healthcare system. (Let the resources be directed to where they are most needed.)
- Practice good hand hygiene, because soap and water can kill Ebola as well as many other more common germs.
- Follow directives from health officials.
- Report relevant exposure history and symptoms to the health department.

Head to www.dummies.com/extras/ebolamythandfacts for more Dummies content online related to Ebola and pregnancy.

In this part . . .

- ✔ Distinguish the similarities and differences between influenza and Ebola symptoms so that you can see how closely related they are.

- ✔ Discover what makes Ebola difficult to catch and understand that people living in the United States, Canada, and Western Europe are at very low risk.

- ✔ Determine whether a patient needs to be isolated, quarantined, or monitored and what each term means.

- ✔ Realize the importance of contact tracing in the efforts to stop an outbreak and how health professionals conduct contact tracing.

Chapter 4

Considering Modes of Transmission and Prevention Methods

In This Chapter

▶ Understanding the ways that Ebola is transmitted

▶ Taking preventative actions — both for yourself and for society

▶ Using protective equipment and following procedures

▶ Knowing when to quarantine, isolate, or self-monitor

*D*uring any sort of public health scare, people usually immedi-ately want to know just how contagious the illness is, whether they can catch it, and how to make sure that they don't. During these times, a lot of misinformation is out there. People don't always have the resources or access to the facts early on, so half-truths, myths, and even downright lies perpetuate. Knowing the facts is important when understanding just how Ebola is transmitted and how you can protect yourself and your loved ones. Educating yourself about this virus helps keep society healthy and emotions in check.

This chapter focuses specifically on the ways that Ebola is trans-mitted and how you as well as society can prevent transmission. You can also find out how healthcare workers in the field keep themselves safe with proper infection prevention and control, and discover the difference between isolation and quarantine.

Seeing How Ebola Is Transmitted

You can contract the Ebola virus only one way — through *direct contact with an infected human or animal's body fluid*. Ebola isn't waterborne or airborne. So far, no evidence suggests that mosquitos carry it. Ebola is spread primarily by *people,* who give it to other people. These sections identify the different ways in which you can come in direct contact with infected body fluids.

Human-to-human contact with body fluids

Living and dead patients infected with Ebola transmit the virus to other people when their body fluids come in direct contact with another person's *mucous membranes* (which are in the eyes, ears, nose, mouth, genitals, and anus) or breaks in the skin. *Direct contact* means that the fluid has gotten into your eyes, nose, mouth, or *non-intact skin* (which can refer to a wound, cut, or even microscopic break in the skin).

The following constitute a *body fluid:*

- ✔ Blood
- ✔ Feces
- ✔ Mucus
- ✔ Saliva
- ✔ Semen
- ✔ Sweat
- ✔ Urine
- ✔ Vomit

On average, most people aren't at risk of contracting Ebola. The people at risk are family members and friends of someone who has had Ebola as well as healthcare workers who have cared for Ebola patients. If you have been or are a healthcare worker who has cared for an Ebola patient, you can take precautions to protect yourself from transmission. (Refer to Chapter 7 for more information.)

Although a case of sexual transmission of Ebola has never been reported, it's technically possible. You should remember this, especially if you're a male or have a male partner who has recovered from Ebola, because the virus can stay in semen for quite some time. Recovered men should abstain from sex (including oral) or use condoms for three months after recovery.

Droplets

Ebola can be transmitted through what are called droplets. *Droplet* transmission refers to large respiratory droplets that are emitted by a cough or sneeze. These droplets travel no more than three feet, and transmission requires prolonged contact with the source patient. Although scientists don't yet know how long it is for Ebola specifically, for other pathogens transmitted by droplets, it equates to hours.

An example of another disease transmitted by droplets is meningococcal meningitis, which, contrary to popular belief, isn't all that contagious, with household transmission rates below 5 percent.

Droplet transmission isn't the same as airborne transmission. The difference is subtle, but important, to remember, because *you can't get Ebola from just sitting in the same room with an infected patient.*

The distinction seems confusing at first, because airborne transmission is referred to as via droplet nuclei. The difference is that one word — *nuclei.* The nuclei are what remain after the droplet has evaporated, and they're what can be transmitted on air currents. They don't even require contact with the source patient. A common example is chickenpox, which has household transmission rates of more than 90 percent if the exposed person isn't immune. Chickenpox nuclei require the high filtration n95 respirator masks to prevent transmission.

Transmission of these *pathogens* (the medical term for anything that can produce disease) can be prevented by wearing a routine surgical mask, hence the initial CDC guidelines for personal protective equipment for Ebola (refer to the later section, "Using personal protective equipment [PPE]" for more details).

Contaminated syringes and medical waste

Contaminated syringes and other medical waste that contain the body fluids of an infected patient can infect you if you touch them. If you're near this material, you should completely avoid it. If you're a healthcare worker who needs to touch it, refer to Chapter 7 and follow all appropriate guidelines regarding safe injection and phlebotomy procedures, including safe management of sharps to dispose of waste properly.

How burial and death rituals can lead to the spread of Ebola

West Africans from different countries — and even different villages and cities within those countries — have beliefs and traditions that differ from one another in how they perceive sickness and death. Here are a few examples that illustrate why Ebola might have spread so quickly in this area:

- Sickness is a punishment that people must serve when they have wronged someone, whether intentional or not. The cure is not medicine (and especially not western medicine); the cure is full confession of all wrongs. If the person dies, it means he didn't confess fully.

- The natural world has an order based on allowing different life forms to be in their own space for reproduction and death (humans should be in their villages, crops in the fields, and animals in the bush), so if a person is very ill, she is to stay home so that she can die there. If she were to die in the bush (perhaps on the way to medical clinic), it brings a curse upon the harvest.

- Pregnant women shouldn't be buried with their fetus still inside them because doing so upsets the order by exposing new life to end of life. If a pregnant woman dies, the fetus must be removed before burial — a process that involves much blood (that is highly infectious, if she has Ebola).

- Relatives of very sick and dying people are obligated to tend to the dying's every wish so she doesn't become angry after death. This anger would result in curses upon the village, which is why many people don't want to take their Ebola-sickened relatives to isolation units. They can't care for them there.

- Immediately after death, the family and relatives gather to wash, oil, and dress the body (which is when most people probably come into contact with Ebola-infected blood and other fluids). The funeral begins right after the person dies, but it can last several days so people from around the area have time to visit. Then they bury the body in their village.

Funeral/burial traditions and other beliefs

A major contributing factor to the outbreak in West Africa is the amount of physical contact that folks have with infected people during local funeral and burial rituals. Typically, in many West African cultures, after someone's death the family of the deceased customarily touches, washes, and kisses the body. Since the late stages of Ebola involve body fluids (refer to the earlier section in this chapter, "Human-to-human contact with body fluids" for specifics), this custom creates immediate exposure to the virus during its most dangerous and contagious time.

Not only are the family members who perform the funeral and burial rituals in direct danger of becoming infected, but anyone who comes into contact with the deceased also is because the deceased often carries residual fluids on their own bodies. Remember, Ebola transmission can happen fast, when one tiny drop of infected blood enters through a tiny (and perhaps invisible) cut in someone's finger without the person even knowing. This is why preventive measures are so important. (Refer to the nearby sidebar for more information about West African death and burial rituals.)

Bush meat

In the United States, Canada, and Western Europe, there is absolutely no threat of Ebola being transmitted through the preparation of food. However, in Africa, people can contract Ebola by hunting, dressing, and butchering infected bush meat (although it's a relatively rare occurrence). Most people who hunt and eat bush meat generally do so without any incident. (Although cooking does kill Ebola, people can contract Ebola when handling and preparing tainted meat.)

Staying away from bush meat is relatively easy for visitors to West Africa, such as healthcare workers, to abide by, but doing so is a bit more challenging for locals who rely on that meat to feed their families.

Taking Precautions to Prevent Contracting Ebola

Most people in the United States, Canada, and Western Europe (and other countries that don't have an active Ebola outbreak) aren't in danger of contracting the virus because of the nature of transmission.

In order to contract Ebola, your mucous membranes or non-intact skin have to come in contact with an infected person's body fluid, either directly (in which case, transmission is very fast) or indirectly via droplet (which takes quite a bit longer).

However, you can still contribute to global prevention efforts. Read on to discover all about the different ways that an individual and society can help to prevent the spread of Ebola.

Travel bans don't work

No matter how temptingly easy they may seem, travel bans don't work. Not only do they border on xenophobia and racism, no pun intended, but they also consider that people originating out of affected areas don't always take direct routes to their destination. So even if a traveler from the affected area has Ebola, he may have had a connection (or several), which means that he could easily enter the country from a non-affected area.

Secondly, isolating the region of the outbreak — allowing no one in or out — would eliminate the ability to freely give and receive humanitarian aid. Some even argue that the United States should bring more patients here so that they can take advantage of the healthcare.

Additionally, sealed borders create illegal (and much more dangerous) crossings. The problem though is that people are still going to cross; the only difference is that they will do it in secret and without safety measures, such as screenings. Without safety measures being followed, there's no telling where the virus could end up. In an area of the world in which borders are porous, those individuals who have the means and the desire to leave only have to walk across the border to enter a country that doesn't have travel restrictions. Many individuals in that area of the world are citizens of more than one country.

Finally, a travel ban encourages people to lie about their itinerary. With porous borders, passports often aren't stamped. When people aren't honest about their travel/exposure history, efforts to control the spread of Ebola can be seriously hampered.

On an individual level

The absolute best way to prevent yourself from contracting and spreading Ebola is simply to avoid outbreak areas and infected people. If you do so, you won't get Ebola.

Here are more prevention tips:

- ✔ **Follow directives from health officials.** Conditions are still changing rapidly, and you never know when something might develop that requires you to listen to and comply with instructions from officials. Although very rare, a possible scenario is that you're notified that one of your contacts has Ebola and you need to be monitored.

- ✔ **Notify health officials if you come into contact with someone who has Ebola.** Again, coming into contact would be rare outside of the affected area, but it's possible. If it happens, call your local health department for guidance.

- ✔ **If you suspect someone in your family or community has Ebola, encourage him to seek help and support him.** Having Ebola-like symptoms in today's climate can be terrifying (on top of the misery of being ill). If someone you know looks like he could have symptoms, make sure that he knows you're going to help and support him. Offer to call the health department for him and let them know that you'll be with him all the way through (as much as is safe).

- ✔ **Although highly discouraged, if you want to care for or have physical contact with someone who has Ebola, notify health officials so that they can train you and give you personal protective equipment (PPE).** In addition to it being a very complex condition to manage and treat, Ebola is highly contagious and requires caregivers to take extreme and fastidious safety measures to ensure the virus isn't passed to them. A medical facility with a trained staff of professionals is the best option for the patient's and your health and well-being. However, if you've made up your mind, you need to learn all that you can to stay safe. (Check out the later section, "Using personal protective equipment [PPE]" for more information about PPEs.)

- ✔ **After visiting someone in the hospital or other facility, wash your hands thoroughly.** Simple soap and water kills most germs (including the Ebola virus), so it's a vital practice if you've been around sick people in general.

- ✔ **Avoid contact with fruit bats, monkeys, and apes in the affected areas.** The exact host animal/s of Ebola are unknown at this time, but bats, monkeys, and apes have all been suspected of carrying it.

- ✔ **Participate fully and be honest and forthright during traveler and medical screenings.** Researchers know that diagnosing and treating Ebola early are key to prevention and recovery (see more in Chapter 5), so if someone asks you about your travel history or any symptoms, just be honest. No one is asking these questions to be nosey or pushy; it's all about staying safe. And who knows — you just may save your own life.

On a society level

Two weapons that a society has against an outbreak like Ebola are an adequate healthcare system and education. An *adequate healthcare system* gives citizens access to quality, affordable, and effective healthcare. Ideally, the system should also have a public health infrastructure, with the capacity to (in this case) rapidly identify patients suspected of having Ebola and to identify and monitor their contacts. *Education* means that a country's citizens are knowledgeable about various aspects of health and safety. As an example of health education working to combat an outbreak, Senegal used a short message service (SMS) to reach its people. Through this campaign, citizens were encouraged to alert health officials if they knew of anyone showing signs of fever and bleeding.

Here are other ways that you can support efforts to ensure the country's healthcare system remains strong and to help other countries develop theirs in the fight against Ebola:

- ✓ **Use your votes to support candidates who support improvements in the public health system and not measures fueled by hysteria over science.** Do your homework and elect people who have had records of voting for and investing in public health improvements, and who will be able to think and act soundly in times of crisis. An example of a solution based on hysteria and not science is enacting travel bans. Refer to the nearby sidebar for why they're not a good idea for preventing Ebola.

- ✓ **Demand that Congress specifically approves funding to help fight Ebola.** The more funding that the United States and other countries can send to the fight, the sooner the fight will be over. Current estimates put the cost of this outbreak at more than $32 billion. A bill is currently in Congress right now, awaiting approval. Contact your representatives and tell them to support it. If Ebola can be stopped in the affected area, then it can be stopped from spreading to the United States.

- ✓ **Donate to organizations that are fighting Ebola in West Africa.** Thousands of volunteers and staff from non-governmental organizations are on the ground and behind the scenes, doing vital response and education work. Without funds to keep going, their efforts will cease. (Flip to Chapter 9 for some ideas about where to donate.)

- ✓ **Educate yourself on the facts so that you don't contribute to hysteria.** You can safely check this one off this list, because you're reading this book.

- ✓ **Get a flu shot so you don't overwhelm the healthcare system.** Let the resources be directed to where they're most needed.

The best way to prevent Ebola from spreading across North America is to get it under control in West Africa. The media's skewed focus on the United States versus West Africa outbreaks is not only inaccurate, but it also can be harmful. The sometimes stigmatizing way society (news media, health officials, even neighbors) treats healthcare workers who go to West Africa and then return (putting them in unnecessary quarantines or even firing them) is having a profound effect on the numbers of volunteers.

For example, the child of a healthcare worker at Bellevue Hospital Center in New York, where one of the United States' Ebola patients was treated, was banned from day care and another one was no longer allowed to go to her usual hairdresser. Individuals who care for patients with Ebola should be praised rather than shunned, and healthcare workers who refuse to care for patients with any disease should be treated the same way as a firefighter who refuses to go into a burning building.

These healthcare workers aren't a danger to the United States. Treating them like pariahs for contributing to humanitarian aid hurts the effort and only prolongs the outbreak, which may lead to more imported cases.

Refer to `www.dummies.com/extras/ebolamythsandfacts` for how to avoid stigmatizing people in this Ebola discussion.

Using Public Education as a Prevention Tool

In addition to treating the current patients, engaging in a robust public education is important and vital. Without the public's buy-in, the epidemic can't stop — and even if did, it wouldn't stay gone. Spreading the word about Ebola is paramount. Here are some ways that the education process is happening in West Africa:

- ✔ **Television and radio:** TV and radio are the fastest and most efficient ways to reach a large amount of people, especially in the urban areas. More people in the affected areas have radios than have TVs. And in the more remote areas, people in the affected areas may not have either, so TV and radio can't be the only method used.

- ✔ **SMS and text messages:** Using technology however possible is important. A unique campaign in Sierra Leone used these short format messages to remind people to wash their hands or report symptoms. It was well received and successful.

- ✔ **Door-to-door visits:** Although some locals receive strangers suspiciously, door-to-door visits are the only way many people can be reached. When someone from the area (versus a foreign volunteer) can do these visits, they're more successful.

- ✔ **Company-sponsored prevention and survivor support:** The Firestone Company made headlines when it initiated its own response effort when an employee's wife was diagnosed with Ebola. The company made treatment available and put tracing, monitoring, and prevention measures in place.

- ✔ **Posters and signage:** Placing messaging where possible in public places helps reinforce the importance and effectiveness of prevention. Many community campaign volunteers also wear messages like "STOP EBOLA" on their clothing.

✔ **Gatherings and meetings:** Community leaders who are well known and respected are typically the key to motivating the masses. They must call together their constituents and friends to help spread the facts.

✔ **Passing out hand-washing supplies and providing instruction:** Going in person to deliver soap, water, chlorine, and buckets, and teaching people how to wash their hands has been a very effective and important public education tool.

Comprehending Special Prevention Measures For Healthcare Workers

Some healthcare workers in affected areas have been infected in nearly every Ebola outbreak since the first one in 1976. Losing healthcare workers to infection has devastating consequences, including the ability to provide services, closures of medical centers, and distrust in the system.

During an outbreak, healthcare workers take specific preventive measures to protect themselves and others in the affected areas, called *standard and other additional precautions.* Following these evidence-based guidelines is imperative for the stoppage of an outbreak. The following sections are meant for the general population only as a basic overview to understand what healthcare workers do. These sections can give you a glimpse of the massive policies and procedures for your own personal understanding. If you're a healthcare worker who is heading into (or already in) the affected area, flip to Chapter 7 for more detailed information.

Identify, isolate, inform

For the general public that may come into contact with Ebola patients, I want to emphasize the simple Centers for Disease Control and Prevention (CDC) procedure of "identify, isolate, inform." If someone is suspected of Ebola, the healthcare worker should place the patient in a room with the door closed and call the local health department.

Doing so is important because many localities have designated receiving hospitals with prepared isolation facilities and trained staff. When the suspected ill patient is identified, he then can be directly transported to an appropriate facility. If the individual is sent directly to an emergency room, further spread may occur before appropriate isolation has been implemented. For more information about what to do if you suspect you or someone you know has Ebola, turn to Chapter 5.

Using personal protective equipment (PPE)

Personal protective equipment (PPE) is all the stuff that healthcare workers put on to protect themselves. When you watch the news, you may have seen the workers covered from head to toe in suits and masks and so on, just like in Figure 4-1. As the outbreak rages on, health officials (mostly at the World Health Organization [WHO] and CDC) continue to tweak procedures for *donning* (putting on) and *doffing* (taking off), amount and type of equipment, and more.

PPE for Ebola currently consists of the following:

- ✓ Powered air purifying respirator (PAPR) or high-filtration mask (n95 respirator).

- ✓ Fluid-resistant medical mask that doesn't collapse against the mouth.

- ✓ Coveralls with single-use disposable hoods.

- ✓ Single-use disposable full-face shields (instead of goggles).

- ✓ Single-use disposable nitrile gloves with extended cuffs (two pairs at the same time). The healthcare worker uses heavy-duty rubber gloves for waste management and environmental cleaning.

- ✓ Single-use disposable fluid-resistant boots that extend to mid-calf.

- ✓ Single-use disposable fluid-resistant or impermeable apron that covers torso to mid-calf if vomit or diarrhea are present.

Healthcare workers are to don and doff PPE in a specific order and under observation. In fact, there are 12 steps for donning and between 20 and 30 for doffing! That gives you a sense of just how intense the protocol is — and why, especially in the early days of the outbreak, protocol can unknowingly be breached, leading to exposure. For the exact steps of what to put on and how to take it off, flip to Chapter 7.

After the disposable items on that list are used, they're removed, placed into temporary secure, fluid-proof bags or containers, and then incinerated. In some instances, they're *autoclaved* (steam cleaned under high pressure) before they're incinerated. The ashes are then disposed of according to local regulations.

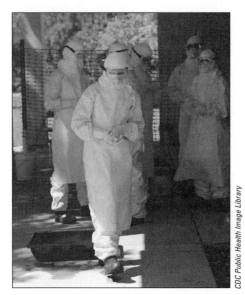

Figure 4-1: Healthcare workers in West Africa wearing their PPE.

Following good hygiene

Hand hygiene is a specific term and is the most effective strategy for preventing the spread of infections, Ebola-affected settings included. Healthcare workers perform hand hygiene with alcohol-based hand sanitizer, soap and water, or, in settings where neither is locally available, a mild (0.05 percent) chlorine solution. Soap and warm water is usually the best option for killing the most germs.

Sanitizer is a good option in an Ebola environment because it kills the virus, is easy to put on, and dries quickly. However, whenever a healthcare worker's hands become visibly soiled with dirt, blood, or body fluids, he needs to use soap and water because sanitizer doesn't work as well when hands are dirty.

Cleaning and maintaining work surfaces

Another key precaution that healthcare workers adhere to is regularly and rigorously cleaning the environment (*environment* refers to the room or ward in which patients with Ebola are cared for), including decontaminating surfaces and equipment. ***Note:*** All approved disinfectant cleaning solutions used in healthcare facilities kill Ebola.

Disposing properly of human remains and medical waste

Human remains and medical waste associated with Ebola are highly contagious, so healthcare workers must handle them according to specific and thorough guidelines. For the purposes of this book, I outline some parts of the major points as examples so you can get a sense of just how involved this process is. This little glimpse of a much larger process (and processes within processes) illustrates why getting Ebola under control is so difficult. And keep in mind, too, that as conditions change, these protocols change. These guidelines are current as of the time of publishing.

Here are the general principles that apply to all healthcare workers in all situations involving remains and medical waste:

- ✔ Only personnel trained in handling infected human remains and wearing PPE should touch or move any Ebola-infected remains.

- ✔ Handling of human remains should be kept to a minimum.

- ✔ Autopsies on patients who die of Ebola should be avoided. If an autopsy is necessary, the state health department and CDC should be consulted regarding additional precautions.

- ✔ Always take into account religious and cultural concerns.

Post-return quarantining, isolating, and monitoring

Three main precautionary methods are used to make sure health-care workers returning to the United States aren't bringing Ebola with them. They are as follows:

- ✔ *Quarantines* are periods of confinement, usually involuntary and mandatory. No one, except for essential medical staff, is in contact with the patient as he is observed and medically monitored for 21 days (the long range of the incubation period for Ebola). Quarantines are applied when the patient has been exposed to Ebola and may or may not become sick.

- ✔ *Isolation* is for people who are known or suspected to have Ebola. The patient is placed in an appropriate facility (I discuss more about these facilities in Chapter 5) for as long as he is symptomatic away from other patients so that he can be treated and not spread it. These isolation wards have their own space, equipment, staff, and protocols.

✔ *Self-monitoring* is also done for 21 days, but it's done at home, where the patient usually can come and go as he pleases as he normally would, as long as he submits to regular monitoring for and reports any symptoms. Dr. Craig Spencer, the doctor in New York was self-monitored. Despite widespread criticism, he was promptly and appropriately isolated and cared for and didn't spread the virus to anyone else prior to being isolated.

The words *quarantine* and *isolation* often get used interchangeably, but they're actually different. Generally speaking, the CDC (and other government and health agencies) doesn't recommend or support mandatory quarantines for healthcare workers coming back from West Africa, unless they're at the highest risk for contracting Ebola. (To be the highest risk, they must have at least four risk categories.) Instead, most workers can self-monitor and report symptoms, if they arise. Some states, however, have taken matters into their own hands.

New York Governor Andrew Cuomo and New Jersey Governor Chris Christie were among those who imposed a mandatory 21-day quarantine for all workers coming back from West Africa, regardless of symptoms (or lack thereof) or risk level. Kaci Hickox, a nurse who came back from serving in Sierra Leone, was forced into quarantine in New Jersey. She fought it and won release to her home state of Maine, where she was also ordered to stay quarantined. She refused and ended up in court. She won and successfully completed a 21-day self-monitoring course at home. What's interesting to note is that she lives with her boyfriend who never contracted Ebola, either.

Quarantines and isolation are obviously vital for infection control when real concerns and threats exist, but when irrational fear — rather than science — is the driving force behind issuing them, it makes for an ineffective health policy and divides the population at a time when it should be pulling together.

Chapter 5

Receiving a Diagnosis and Undergoing Treatment

*I*dentifying and diagnosing Ebola in a person who has been infected for only a few days is difficult because the early symptoms are so common. The symptoms are easily confused with the flu (as well as malaria and typhoid in Africa).

However, the key is this: If a person has the early symptoms of Ebola *plus* has had contact with body fluids of an Ebola patient, objects that have been contaminated with body fluids of an Ebola patient, or Ebola-infected animals, you may have a problem. A big one.

This chapter identifies the symptoms of Ebola (which you can see are similar to other common ailments), takes you through what to do if you as a civilian encounter someone who you think has Ebola, explains how Ebola is actually tested for, gives you a rundown of the various experimental drugs and treatments right now, and examines what happens during the recovery process.

Recognizing the Symptoms

If you're exposed to Ebola, it can take anywhere from 2 to 21 days for you to start showing symptoms, with the average being 8 to 10 days (this is known as the *incubation period*). Ebola has two stages of symptoms as the virus progresses. Symptoms in the first stage are quite flulike, starting with any (probably several) of the following:

- Fever greater than 101.5 degrees
- Weakness
- Muscle pain
- Headache
- Lack of appetite
- Sore throat

Then the symptoms progress to more severe:

- Rash
- Diarrhea
- Vomiting
- Unexplained bleeding or bruising
- Impaired liver and kidney function

A person isn't contagious unless and until she actually shows symptoms of Ebola. Patients that are in the later stage of Ebola are more contagious than those patients in the earlier stage. Because Ebola shares a lot of symptoms with the flu, it's good to compare the differences between the two viruses, as Table 5-1 outlines.

Table 5-1   The Differences Between the Flu and Ebola

Flu	*Ebola*
Symptoms usually appear within 2 days of exposure.	Symptoms can appear anywhere from 2 to 21 days after exposure.
Symptoms come on quickly, all at once.	Symptoms develop over several days and gradually increase in severity.
Fever and headache	Fever and severe headache
Cough	Muscle pain
Sore throat	Fatigue and weakness
Runny or stuffy nose	Vomiting and diarrhea start after three to six days.
	Stomach pain
	Unexplained bruising or bleeding

Knowing What to Do If You Think You or Someone Has Ebola

If you suspect that you or someone else has Ebola, and you're in the United States, Canada, or Western Europe, don't panic. Remember, Ebola is very rare to contract in these countries. But still, you should move swiftly.

If you're in one of the affected areas (in West Africa), then the situation is a bit direr and requires absolute urgent attention. Stick to these steps:

1. **Ask if the person has lived in or traveled to an affected area or come into contact with a confirmed Ebola patient in the last 21 days.**

   If you suspect that you're ill, ask yourself the same questions. If not, it's highly unlikely that you or this person has Ebola (assuming she is being honest and has full knowledge of her contacts). If the answer is yes (or there's any doubt), proceed to the next step.

2. **Identify signs and symptoms.**

   Do you or the person have fever (subjective or greater or equal to 100.4 degrees F or 38 degrees C) or do you or the person have Ebola-like symptoms (refer to the earlier section in this chapter, "Recognizing the Symptoms" for specifics)? If no, then you or the person probably doesn't have Ebola. If yes (or if you're in doubt), proceed to the next step.

3. **Isolate.**

   Place yourself or the person in an isolated room and close the door and then call the health department. The health professionals will instruct you about what to do. You may even want to put some sort of signage on the door, if needed, to inform others.

If you're traveling and you suspect someone has Ebola, alert airline (or whatever mode of transportation you're using) staff. Those personnel have a protocol to follow regarding those situations. They're supposed to ask any sick travelers if they have been in Guinea, Liberia, or Sierra Leone in the past 21 days. If the answer is no, they follow their routine procedures. If the answer is yes and the symptoms are consistent with Ebola, they're supposed to report it immediately to the CDC, and they may separate the passenger from others.

Naming the hospitals that can handle Ebola

The United States has four *biocontainment units,* which are units within bigger facilities, designed to treat the most contagious and virulent illnesses that afflict humans. Their staffs are highly trained and practiced on very specific infection prevention protocols. They're funded by the government and meant to keep one infection from becoming an epidemic, so as Ebola patients are evacuated to or discovered in the United States, they can end up in one of these four locations:

✔ Emory University Hospital in Atlanta, Georgia

✔ National Institutes of Health in Bethesda, Maryland

✔ University of Nebraska Medical Center in Omaha, Nebraska

✔ St. Patrick Hospital in Missoula, Montana

These highly specialized units have been designed with many different infection prevention and control features, among them:

✔ **Negative airflow:** Clean, filtered air comes in without letting the contaminated air out.

✔ **Windows and intercoms:** Nurses can interact with patients without having to don all of their protective equipment.

✔ **Waste protocols:** At Emory, disposable goods are first pressure-steamed, and then incinerated. Body fluids (such as urine) are treated for at least five minutes with bleach or detergent before being flushed.

✔ **Biopods:** Also called *isopods,* they are giant containment umbrellas or bubbles that fit tightly over gurneys so that staff can take someone from outside into the isolation ward safely.

Since the risk of spreading Ebola is low, even in an airplane (because Ebola isn't airborne; refer to Chapter 4 for ways that Ebola is transmitted), the pilots don't have to do anything like emergency land the plane. Crew members just follow their infection control guidelines until the plane lands and then notify ground crews and other personnel as needed.

Identifying Everyone with Whom the Patient Has Had Contact

After a suspected Ebola patient is isolated, healthcare workers commence *contact tracing,* which is the process of finding everyone who has come in direct contact with that patient. Contacts are then watched for signs of illness for 21 days from the last day they came in contact with the Ebola patient.

If the contact never shows symptoms over the course of the 21 days, the contact is declared free and clear of Ebola. If the contact develops a fever or other Ebola symptoms, healthcare workers then bring the patient to a proper healthcare facility to isolate, test, and provide her care. Then the cycle starts again — all of the new patient's contacts are found and watched for 21 days.

Contact tracing finds new cases quickly so that they can be isolated, stopping further spread of Ebola. Figure 5-1 illustrates the process.

Currently, no federal law requires adherence to this process, but states and local jurisdictions are empowered to create and enforce their own, so penalties for not complying vary from state to state. For more information on isolation and how different states have enforced it, turn to Chapter 4.

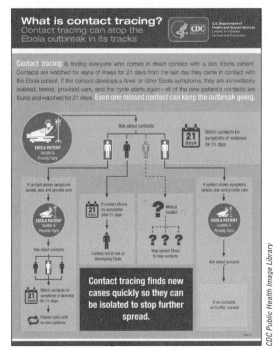

CDC Public Health Image Library

Figure 5-1: Contact tracing is an important part of diagnosis, treatment, and prevention.

Testing and Diagnosing

The good news is that a number of tests, which the following sections identify, can be used to diagnose Ebola within a few days of the onset of symptoms by detecting both the virus and the antibodies to it. The sort of bad news is that it can take several days for some of these tests actually to register as positive, even if the patient does have Ebola, because at first, the virus lives in a person's organs. It takes awhile for the virus to grow enough to get into the blood, which is why isolation during this time is very important.

Polymerase chain reaction test

The most accurate of the tests is the *polymerase chain reaction (PCR)* test, which searches for the tiniest bit of genetic material from the virus and replicates it. Sounds crazy, right? But it replicates the virus so that it can detect it. Otherwise, it can be too tiny to register and could progress under the radar.

The one concern is that this test can be negative during the first three days an infected person has symptoms, so the patient will have to be kept isolated, even if she registers a negative at first. This test is also used to determine when a recovered patient can be discharged.

The unintended consequences on the fight against malaria

The Guinean government reports that the Ebola outbreak has seriously compromised the fight against malaria. Doctors are confusing malaria with Ebola, delaying the right life-saving treatment. Guinea's government committee against malaria said many of the undocumented deaths suspected of being from Ebola may actually be from malaria.

Each year, malaria affects 5 million people and kills at least 10 people in Guinea every week. Compare that to the Ebola outbreak: It began in Guinea in December 2013, has infected fewer than 2,000 people, and caused close to 1,200 deaths. What officials are seeing now is that people are so afraid of being diagnosed with Ebola that they're staying away from medical care, and given that Ebola and malaria share so many symptoms, this is a problem both from an empirical and reporting standpoint as well as a humanitarian one. Lives that could be saved aren't, and all the progress that Guinea has made in its fight against malaria is backsliding.

Antigen-capture enzyme-linked immunosorbent assay

Another test looks for the antibodies produced by the body's immune system in response to the virus. Known as the *antigen-capture enzyme-linked immunosorbent assay (ELISA)*, this test can take even longer than three days to give a positive result for an infected person. The other tricky thing is that, in general, tests can still detect antibodies after a patient recovers, which is why positive tests for things like Lyme disease may only indicate past infection.

If a patient is diagnosed with Ebola, scientists may want to try to isolate and culture the virus so that they can study it. But culturing Ebola is very dangerous, so it's only done in a BSL-4 lab (flip to Chapter 2 to see a list of these labs).

Other testing that might be helpful in diagnosing Ebola include

✔ **Basic blood tests:** Some of these basic blood tests are

- **Complete blood count (CBC) with differential:** This test looks at the white blood cell (or *leukocyte*) count, as well as the red blood cell and platelet counts. The white blood cell count is high for many infections, but can be low in Ebola, which is part of the immune system dysfunction that occurs with this infection. Also, patients can have anemia, and the platelet count may be low. The latter contributes to the bleeding that may be present in patients with Ebola.

- **Bilirubin:** This test can indicate liver problems or breaking open of red blood cells.

- **Liver enzymes, blood urea nitrogen (BUN), and creatinine:** They're indicators of kidney function.

- **pH:** If not enough blood is going to all parts of the body, as occurs in shock, the blood can become *acidic,* which means that the pH will be low.

✔ **Other studies:** Doctors may perform immunochemical testing of postmortem skin and use an electron microscope to look for the virus itself.

In addition to testing for Ebola, doctors also test for related illnesses (which are much more likely to be the cause of symptoms) such as:

Flu, malaria, lassa fever, typhoid fever, meningitis

Figuring Out the Politics behind Vaccines

Currently, no approved vaccines are available for Ebola, which is pretty tragic, considering the current outbreak the world faces. And to add insult to injury, further consider that scientists from the United States and Canada reported in 2005 that they had created one that was 100 percent effective in animal testing and that it could be ready for licensing by 2011. Had that happened, West Africa probably wouldn't be facing the decimation it is now. So what happened?

Some say the delay in moving the vaccine forward happened because Ebola is such a rare disease that only affects a few hundred people at a time (well, until now). Others surmise (and some experts even acknowledge) the delay is because Ebola afflicts poor countries — countries where pharmaceutical companies can't make the money they want off of it. But now that Ebola has been seen in the United States and other non-African countries, the momentum for approving a vaccine has quickened.

All sorts of efforts and funding sources are being worked on now. Two vaccines in North America are currently in human clinical trials, which makes them the furthest along and closest to becoming available (assuming the trials go well):

- ✔ **cAd3-EBOZ:** The University of Maryland is developing this vaccine. It's based on an Ebola virus from a chimpanzee, and it looks to be generating a good antibody response in patients so far.

- ✔ **VSV-EBOV:** The Public Health Agency of Canada's National Microbiology Laboratory in Nova Scotia is developing this vaccine. It's based on an Ebola virus from a cow. In addition to acting as a vaccine, there are signs that it may also help those who already have Ebola.

Researchers from both groups say they should have information about the safety and dosage of the drugs in early January 2015.

The fast tracking of this vaccine development wouldn't be possible without key funding sources, such as:

- ✔ The Canadian government, which has committed $20.7 million for vaccine research and development

✔ The EU's Innovative Medicines Initiative, which has offered up to $350 million for vaccine research and development

✔ The US Congress, which is currently considering a bill for $6.2 billion in total Ebola aid (including research and development), on top of the $423 million already donated and pledged

Considering Treatments

Because Ebola has no cure, the majority of treatment for Ebola is prevention of organ damage and supportive care for the immune system so it can mount an attack on the virus. In addition, some experimental treatments are being used to treat Ebola. These sections examine the different types of treatment — first the standard therapies and then the experimental ones.

Seeing the standard treatment

This treatment includes working to prevent intravascular volume depletion, correcting severe electrolyte imbalances, and avoiding the complications of shock that can come with these complications.

Patients can lose large amounts of fluid through sweating, vomiting, and diarrhea, requiring rapid volume replacement in order to prevent shock. Paying careful attention to fluid losses and intake is a foundational part of the treatment for Ebola. Patients often need IVs to stay hydrated. If they're a little more stable or they respond well to anti-nausea and anti-diarrhea meds, they can orally drink the fluids they need.

Additional supportive measures may include

✔ **Management of fever, nausea, vomiting, diarrhea, and abdominal, joint, and muscle pain:** Contrary to popular belief, fever impairs the growth of many viruses and enhances the immune response. Therefore, it shouldn't be treated unless it's extremely high or directly causing significant discomfort.

✔ **Use of blood products:** These blood products, such as packed red blood cells, platelets, and fresh frozen plasma, are used to treat *coagulopathy* (the reduced ability of the blood to clot) and anemia.

✔ **Renal replacement therapy:** It helps manage renal failure in the setting of shock. Ebola can result in multi-organ failure, and it's not unusual for the kidneys to shut down in later stages of the illness without intervention, so dialysis is often warranted. If the kidneys experience reduced renal function, they may respond to simple fluid replacement, whereas if they are in renal failure, they require dialysis. If dialysis is required, clinicians should refer to the CDC document on how to safely perform acute hemodialysis in patients with Ebola virus disease. Without dialysis, kidney failure can be fatal.

✔ **Oxygen therapy and ventilator support:** Although breathing problems aren't typically associated with Ebola virus disease, *pulmonary edema* (fluid build-up in the lungs) can occur due to the aggressive fluid replacement that Ebola patients need. Among other things, oxygen is often used as part of the treatment for pulmonary edema. Patients may also experience *acute respiratory distress syndrome* or *ARDS* (a severe lung inflammation) due to shock and multi-organ dysfunction. Physicians may treat these conditions with *mechanical ventilation,* which requires that a tube be placed through the mouth into the trachea, which is the large breathing passage to the lungs. The tube is then connected to a machine that provides oxygen and breathes for the patient.

✔ **Blood pressure support:** In Ebola patients, *hypotension* (low blood pressure) is due to the fluid losses. Treatment with oral or IV fluid replacement is often effective, and medications may also be used to increase blood pressure.

✔ **Treatment of other infections, if they occur:** As patients recover from Ebola, the immune system dysfunction caused by this virus can make the patient more likely to get other infections. Monitoring the patient closely for the development of other infections and treating these infections as soon as they occur are important.

Ebola patients must also have intensive nursing monitoring because their condition can change so rapidly.

Eyeing the experimental treatment

Currently, several different treatments are being used experimentally during this outbreak in West Africa. These treatments include the following:

✔ **Antibody preparations:** *Antibodies* are proteins found in the blood that are produced by the body in response to an infection. The antibodies attach to the germs, and in so doing alert the immune system to kill these invaders. (I explain more about this in Chapter 2.) Unfortunately, it can take time for the body to produce enough antibody to fight off an infection, allowing the germ to cause havoc meanwhile. Treatment with antibodies (also known as *immune globulin* or *gamma globulin*) can help the body fight off an infection. Two types of experimental antibody preparations are being used for Ebola:

- **ZMapp:** This is a brand-name drug being developed by a pharmaceutical company called Mapp Biopharmaceutical. It's a mix of three antibodies (that are made by using genetically modified tobacco) aimed at the Ebola viral glycoprotein. These antibodies came out of two existing cocktails called MB-003 and ZMab. It has been given to several patients, including two US healthcare workers, both who survived and recovered. Two other severely ill healthcare workers given ZMapp didn't survive, possibly due to the fact that they received it relatively late in the disease's progression. (Refer to the nearby sidebar for more details about ZMapp.)

- **Serum:** The liquid component of blood, which contains antibodies, but not red cells, white cells, or platelets, from an Ebola survivor is injected into an Ebola patient, presumably so the antibodies in the survivor's blood can help the current patient fight off the infection. Scientists don't know a lot about this treatment yet, because they haven't been able to study it at length. They used blood plasma from a survivor to treat an Ebola patient for the first time in 1976. The patient died, but she had less bleeding than is typical. Since then, only an additional handful of patients have received this treatment, with mixed results (although most patients saw an improvement or survived). This treatment is considered promising and scientists are conducting more research around it. The Institute of Tropical Medicine in Belgium commenced human trials in December 2014, which will last for a year.

✔ **Novel (new) antiviral agents:** These medications act directly against the virus by attacking parts of the virus that are essential for it to reproduce but aren't found in the human body. In so doing, antiviral agents kill the virus but not have any significant effect on our cells. Because viruses must enter cells to reproduce, finding medications that work on them without affecting the patient is difficult, which is why so few effective treatments for viral infections are available. Brincidofovir is a novel antiviral agent and has been reported to have *in vitro* (in the laboratory) activity against the Ebola virus, which is very promising.

✔ **Interfering ribonucleic acid (RNA) particles:** RNA is a molecule that is responsible for genetic coding in the manufacture of proteins, which are essential for all forms of life. Interfering RNA particles can essentially prevent certain expressions of genes, resulting in the production of defective proteins or even no proteins at all. In the case of Ebola, these particles interfere with and break down the glycoproteins, preventing the virus from invading and spreading. Here are a couple of RNA particle experimental treatments:

  • **TKM-Ebola:** It's an RNA interference agent that stops the production of Ebola proteins. In January 2014, it went into the first round of human trials, but then the FDA halted it in July because of side effects. After the Ebola outbreak was declared, the FDA allowed the drug to be used for patients in West Africa, and the full development of this drug is now being expedited.

  • **Antisense phosphorodiamidate morpholino oligomer:** It also interferes with the proteins that Ebola uses to replicate and spread itself. It's still in development, awaiting human clinical trials.

Examining the ZMapp controversy

When ZMapp appeared, the question then became whether any humans should get the drug, given that it hadn't been tested on people yet. And then, after that, the question was: Who exactly should get the limited doses?

In July 2014, Sheik Umar Khan, the African doctor who led the fight against Ebola in Sierra Leone, became infected with Ebola. Even though ZMapp existed, Doctors Without Borders and the World Health Organization (WHO) decided that administering the drug was too risky, and unfortunately Khan died. However, American workers in Liberia contracted Ebola soon afterward, and the remaining dosage of ZMapp was shipped to them instead. A different treatment group decided to administer the drug to the American workers, and they ended up surviving. For many people, this seemingly double standard resulted in loss of life and was enraging and unacceptable. But for others, the issue wasn't cut and dry.

Was this racism, plain and simple? Or was something different at play?

On one hand, you don't want to deny people the chance to live, but on the other hand, you don't want to exploit people by using them as test subjects. In life-threatening emergencies, skipping some clinical testing for drugs may be ethical as long as the patients who are in line to receive the treatment are informed of the risk and consent to treatment. Given that they're facing possible or certain death anyway, many patients would probably love to have the option.

Now onto the next issue: If there was a limited supply, who should be the first to receive it (or receive it at all)? Why did these American workers get it, while Dr. Khan didn't? Weighing the risks and benefits, trying to put a value on a human life, and comprehending the societal implications of deciding who gets treatment and who doesn't is very complex.

Part of the complexity comes from taking into account that early access to treatment is one of the major factors in successful recovery. Some contend that those who can do the most good for the epidemic (like healthcare workers and Dr. Kahn)

should be given priority over common people. Others think people in early stages of the illness should be given priority over people in later stages because they have more of a chance to recover.

The ZMapp controversy has brought to the surface some terrifying life-or-death manifestation of age-old dynamics: rich versus poor, haves versus have-nots, western civilization versus developing countries. These ongoing dichotomies won't be solved now — maybe not ever — but in order to successfully overcome Ebola, the global community has to get a handle on what's really interfering with saving lives.

Recovering from Ebola

Doctors and researchers don't know a lot about Ebola, including why some people recover and other don't. They're starting to get some good ideas, though. For example, they know successful recovery depends on good supportive care and the patient's immune response.

Some of the doctors reporting in from West Africa as they work with Doctors Without Borders say that quick diagnosis and treatment seems also to play a role in how well a patient recovers. If a patient can get in early and get treated (even in West Africa), she has a much better chance of survival. The problem in West Africa is the sheer numbers. West African hospitals don't have enough beds, and the ones they do have go to the sickest patients, which means there just isn't room for people to get in early.

Another issue is that many patients in West Africa have to be treated in the field, in their homes, which means there is no access to all of those supportive treatments and therapies, like IVs.

Some other reports say the manner of transmission may also impact recovery. For example, needlestick cases seem to do worse than those who were infected via mucus membranes.

Individuals who no longer have signs and symptoms of Ebola virus disease can be discharged if they have two negative PCR tests on whole blood, separated by at least 48 hours. (Check out the earlier section, "Polymerase chain reaction [PCR] test" for how this test works.)

Recovering from Ebola depends on factors such as the age and immune status of the patient, severity of illness, what treatment is given, and when it was initiated. The cases in the United States have seemed to last somewhere in the two- to three-week range (go to Chapter 3 for a list of those cases).

People who recover from Ebola develop antibodies that last for at least ten years, possibly longer. Researchers don't yet know if people who recover are immune for life or if they can become infected with a different species of Ebola. Researchers do know that some people who have recovered from Ebola have developed long-term complications, such as joint and vision problems.

Preparing for Post-Ebola Life

Doctors don't yet know a lot about the long-term effects of surviving Ebola, but they do know many survivors suffer from health problems post-recovery. Sometimes called *post-Ebola syndrome,* here are some of the afflictions associated with Ebola survival that doctors have discovered:

- ✔ The virus stays in semen and breast milk for up to three months.
- ✔ Extreme fatigue.
- ✔ *Arthralgia,* a type of joint pain that's similar to arthritis, but without the joint swelling and damage.
- ✔ *Uvetitis,* which is an inflammation that can cause excess tearing, eye sensitivity, eye inflammation, blurred vision, floating spots in the vision, eye pain, redness, and sensitivity to light. In some cases, it can go away in a few days or weeks with treatment (although relapses are common). In other cases, it can last for months or years and may cause permanent impairment or blindness, even with treatment.
- ✔ Damage to kidneys, liver, heart, and long-term fertility issues (as is the case in patients of any severe viral infection).

As for the actual cause(s) of these conditions, doctors are still trying to figure out whether it's actually the disease itself, the treatments, or maybe something in or related to the intense disinfection procedures — or maybe a combination of everything.

Part III

Looking at Today and into the Future

How much the world has given

Country	Donated	Pledged
United States	$206.5 million	$65.6 million
United Kingdom	$18.7 million	$191.5 million
Germany	$16.7million	
Australia	$13.8 million	
Japan	$11.4 million	$32.5 million
Sweden	$11.2 million	$4.3 million
China	$8.2 million	$34 million
France	$7.4 million	
Switzerland	$6.8 million	
Kuwait	$5 million	
Venezuela	$5 million	

Go to www.dummies.com/extras/ebolamythsandfacts for ways to fight the stigma about Ebola.

In this part . . .

- ✔ Analyze the reasons why humanitarian aid for the current outbreak is important and why it has been delayed.

- ✔ Uncover Cuba's special diplomacy in the outbreak response and why Cuba has focused on providing help to many of the world's recent crises.

- ✔ Discover why some healthcare workers in the affected area have been on strike and what it means to having qualified personnel available for the ill.

- ✔ Find out who is caring for the orphans of the outbreak and what you can do if you want to help.

Chapter 6

Eyeing the Geopolitical Outlook and Impact

. . . .

In This Chapter

▶ Examining the reasons behind the delay in response to the 2014 outbreak

▶ Seeing how much funding the world is giving to fight the 2014 and future outbreaks

▶ Understanding the global impact of the 2014 outbreak

. . . .

*A*lthough Ebola was discovered in 1976, with scientists studying and aid organizations tending to outbreaks since, the 2014 outbreak has pushed the disease to the forefront of most discussions on healthcare happening around the world like never before. As the disease bears down on West Africa, it has also affected other countries, but to a much-lesser degree. Still, the reach of this outbreak has been enough to set off a global response (though, some argue, a response that was much too slow to start).

Many layers comprise this response, from politics to culture to race relations. World health leaders, politicians, and scientists have been faced with some tough questions, tough problems, and no easy answers. This chapter (and book) presents a unique opportunity to record a snapshot of the world as it stands now. I hope that they can make enough progress soon to halt Ebola once and for all. Then work can focus on ensuring it never happens again.

Criticizing the WHO's Response to the 2014 Outbreak

Although they are considered the world leader for international public health, the World Health Organization (WHO) has been widely criticized for its slow recognition of and response to the

2014 Ebola outbreak. To set the stage, here is the timeline of the early events:

- **March 22:** Guinea identifies a hemorrhagic fever that killed 50 people as Ebola.

- **March 30:** Liberia reports two Ebola cases. Sierra Leone reports that it thinks it might have Ebola cases as well.

- **April 1:** Doctors Without Borders, already providing care in the area, warns WHO that there is a dangerous and unprecedented outbreak afoot. WHO doesn't agree with the assessment at that time.

- **May 26:** WHO confirms the first Ebola deaths in Sierra Leone.

- **June 23:** Doctors Without Borders says the outbreak is out of control and makes a call for immediate mass response and resources.

- **July 2–3:** WHO convenes a subregional emergency meeting in Ghana to discuss and plan a response to the outbreak.

- **July 21–25:** WHO's regional director visits the affected countries.

- **July 30:** Liberia shutters schools and imposes mass quarantines.

- **July 31:** WHO and the countries affected in West Africa announce that it will take $100 million in aid to contain the outbreak.

- **August 8:** WHO declares the outbreak an international health emergency.

- **August 11:** WHO's revised guidelines on how to prevent the spread of the disease are released, updating guidelines from 2008.

- **August 12:** WHO announces the death toll tops 1,000 and approves use of experimental drugs and vaccines.

- **August 28:** WHO publishes a road map to guide and coordinate the international response to the outbreak, aiming to stop the epidemic in six to nine months. WHO simultaneously revises its cost estimate for the next six months to $490 million.

  Other than cases in which individuals are suspected or have been confirmed of being infected with Ebola or have had contact with cases of Ebola, WHO doesn't recommend any travel or trade restrictions.

In response, WHO says that Ebola had been bad in Central Africa, but had never been seen before in West Africa, so officials weren't on the lookout for it. And when WHO finally declared the outbreak an international public health emergency in August, WHO says its declaration wasn't made strongly or loudly enough in order to create a sense of understanding and urgency among world health leaders. WHO admits it could've done more to sound the alarm bell and organize colleagues.

Up until about this point in time, WHO defended itself and its response, but then an internal report surfaced in mid-October that confirmed the world's assessment. Some of the issues mentioned in the report include

- ✔ WHO experts in the field failed to send reports to WHO headquarters.
- ✔ Red tape prevented $500,000 from reaching the response effort in Guinea.
- ✔ Doctors were unable to gain access to affected areas because visas hadn't been obtained.

WHO also points to budget problems, saying that it hadn't increased dues in more than a decade, leading to shortfalls and gaps. Private donors, who all have their own interests and ear-marks, had to fill those shortfalls, which meant that when there was something unexpected (like an unprecedented West African Ebola outbreak), no money was available to handle it. To put a number on it, WHO's annual spending is $2 billion, which is less than some US hospitals' spending!

Priorities also shifted among members of WHO from disease identi-fication and response to treatment and prevention of illnesses and ailments like heart disease and obesity. Even the more impover-ished nations shifted, suggesting that the well-off representatives had lost touch with their poverty-stricken citizens. In 2011, they all voted down a proposal for a $100 million epidemic taskforce.

Some also suggest that WHO's regional office in Africa failed to properly monitor West Africa's Ebola outbreak, given that it began in December, but the first cases weren't reported until March.

Looking At the UN Mission for Ebola Emergency Response

The UN Security Council declared the outbreak a threat to interna-tional peace and security and unanimously adopted United Nations Security Council Resolution 2177, a temporary initiative to increase immediate aid to and crisis management in the affected areas (in addition to what the WHO was already doing). This unprecedented initiative is now called the United Nations Mission for Ebola Emergency Response (UNMEER), and its main task is coordinating the UN's resources under the leadership of WHO.

UNMEER now works closely with governments; regional and international actors, such as the African Union (AU) and the Economic Community of West African States (ECOWAS); the private sector; and civil society. Accra, Ghana, is serving as a base for UNMEER, and the UNMEER has teams in Guinea, Liberia, and Sierra Leone.

This initiative has five goals that will cost approximately $1 billion to implement and manage. They are

- ✔ Stop the outbreak
- ✔ Treat the infected
- ✔ Ensure essential services
- ✔ Preserve stability
- ✔ Prevent outbreaks

Examining CDC's Response

Despite early criticisms (most from Republicans during a Congressional hearing in October) that it didn't provide accurate and adequate Ebola prevention information, the CDC has generally received praise for its actions.

Currently, it runs the Ebola Emergency Operations Center, which is one of the main coordinating bodies. From that, it deploys and manages hundreds of staff and experts in the affected areas, the countries that border the affected areas, and in the United States. The CDC teams provide much of the operational infrastructure through contact tracing, surveillance, data management, and more.

It has also created and is managing the guidelines and information regarding travel screening, procedures for airlines, and border management, and is working with the hospitals in the United States to make sure they are prepared for Ebola patients.

Understand Why Humanitarian Aid Has Been Delayed

Aside from the seeming late initiation of leadership from WHO, one of the main reasons why there was a delay in the time it took for countries to come to the aid of West Africa is because they were busy putting protective and preventive measures in place for their own countries, such as:

✔ Sending out travel advisory notices to warn of the potential risk of travel to countries affected by the epidemic

✔ Withholding visitor visas from people in the affected countries, closing borders, cancelling flights, and stopping ship arrivals

✔ Implementing initiatives such as creating isolation facilities, training staff, conducting biocontainment exercises, launching notification hotlines, stockpiling drugs and equipment, and performing health screenings on incoming travellers

As the outbreak has gone on, world leaders have stepped up, and nations from around the globe have come together to offer aid in various forms. Currently, Ebola is under control everywhere except West Africa, and current forecasts suggest a change in the outbreak curve won't happen until the beginning of next year, but at least world powers are finally uniting to stop the outbreak. The general consensus among most world health leaders is that efforts and resources must stay focused on and flowing to the countries of West Africa. They need help from the global health community in order to stop the outbreak and therefore prevent Ebola from continuing to spread into other countries.

Humanitarian aid comes in all forms: funding, personnel, supplies, education and outreach, and more. All types of aid are needed to fight the outbreak successfully. These sections provide a rundown of some of the major types of aid that are currently funneling into West Africa.

Funding

Funding for the West African Ebola outbreak battle got off to a very slow start. The UN made a call in September for countries to contribute $1 billion, but by October, only a third had been raised. Some of the first countries to contribute were the United States, Cuba, and the United Kingdom. Many other countries were still too focused on their own people.

By the end of 2014, the focus has solidly shifted, and countries were not only funneling their own funds to West Africa, but they also were publicly advocating that others do the same. Table 6-1 outlines how much each country has donated (and pledged) to the efforts by December, 2014.

Table 6-1	How Much the World Has Given	
Country	*Donated*	*Pledged*
United States	$206.5 million	$65.6 million
United Kingdom	$18.7 million	$191.5 million
Germany	$16.7million	
Australia	$13.8 million	
Japan	$11.4 million	$32.5 million
Sweden	$11.2 million	$4.3 million
China	$8.2 million	$34 million
France	$7.4 million	
Switzerland	$6.8 million	
Kuwait	$5 million	
Venezuela	$5 million	

Other entities and their contributions include

- The African Development Bank has contributed more than $220 million.
- The Economic Community of West African States (ECOWAS) disbursed $250,000.
- In response to the ECOWAS Special Fund for the Fight Against Ebola, the Nigerian government donated $3.5 million.
- The European Council announced that contributions by the European Commission and individual member states come to a combined total of $1.3 billion.
- The World Bank Group has pledged $500 million.
- Bill and Melinda Gates Foundation has donated $13.6 million and pledged $36.3 million more.

Healthcare workers

Having qualified healthcare workers is one of the greatest needs. Because West Africa doesn't have the advanced healthcare system or even basic societal infrastructure that is needed to combat and prevent a disease like Ebola, medical help from other countries has been vital. Without it, containing this outbreak would be almost hopeless. Various governments and nongovernmental organizations (NGOs) have responded and are working together to give care and stop the spread of the virus. These sections highlight two examples.

Cuba: A (not so) surprising leader

Healthcare professionals from all over the world have responded to the emergency, although the first country out of the gate to respond was — believe it or not — Cuba.

On September 12, 2014, President Raúl Castro's health minister announced that Cuba would send nearly 500 healthcare professionals to West Africa. Since then, 165 have arrived in Sierra Leone and 83 in Liberia and Guinea (with 200 more expected). This amount is the most healthcare workers any country or organization has sent, even counting Doctors Without Borders.

Cuba is known for its mobile medical teams and has become quite the world's first responder to international crises in recent years, such as the Pakistan earthquake in 2005 and the 2010 Haiti earthquake. More than 50,000 Cuban medical workers are estimated to be helping in areas of most need around the world.

This assistance is the result of a long-term strategy that the Cuban government has pursued since taking power in 1959, and it's both economic and political. Healthcare workers are an exportable resource that they can produce on a large scale. And it's paid off for Cuba in big ways — to the tune of $8 billion annually. And Cuba's reputation as a medical powerhouse has also set up Cuba as a more respected country and destination for medical training.

Aside from actually saving lives, this move has political implications, most notably between Cuba and the United States and Cuba and the United Nations. US and UN leaders have publicly praised Cuba's Ebola efforts and considered it a very positive thing to be working side-by-side with them.

Healthcare Workers' Rights Movement: Standing up for workers

Participation in the Ebola outbreak by medical professionals hasn't all been about goodwill, however. Many healthcare workers (especially in the beginning of the outbreak) contracted the virus and died, which were the stories shown on the news. The rampant media coverage of these deaths created a fear among healthcare workers. They're reluctant to go help, for fear of their own health and lives. And for those who are there now, staying safe while caring for patients has become a workers' rights issue.

On October 13, 2014, Liberian nurses threatened to strike, demanding more pay for working in hazardous conditions and to receive better protective gear. The union accused the Liberian government of intimidating workers to return to their jobs. The Monrovian government came out against a strike, saying a strike would be absolutely devastating for the patients who are in dire need.

Then on November 11 and 12, US nurses — first in California and then across several states — protested and went on strike to draw attention to the West Africa plight and to demand better and more protective gear and equipment for hospitals that might encounter possible Ebola patients. Kaiser-Permanente, the hospital system that operates most of the locations where the nurses protested, accused the union of trumping up an excuse for labor action.

Regardless of the outcomes of the strikes, hospitals and governments have to protect their healthcare workers if they want these professionals to keep providing life-saving care.

Other volunteers

In addition to healthcare workers, this outbreak is benefitting from and needs help from all sorts of different professionals. Many terms of service are in the three-to-six-month range, but can be much longer, depending on the agency and the needs of the affected area. Some of the volunteer needs are

Community advocates, public health specialists, nutritionists medical logisticians, field crisis managers, data collectors and managers.

Mobile labs/mini hospitals

Another important part of the humanitarian effort is the donation, construction, and management of mobile labs and mini hospitals. Although a lot of the outbreak is centered in urban areas, plenty of cases are still in the outlying, more remote areas of these countries. Being able to bring the proper diagnostic and treatment equipment to the people is the only way to really get a handle on the outbreak.

Food and supplies

Donations of cash are helpful, and so are donations of food and supplies (like this donation of whole blood that's going to Liberia, pictured in Figure 6-1), which can sometimes be easier for a government, business, or organization to provide. Aside from being directly beneficial to the front lines, donations like these can give the donors a little more mileage than cash, because their logo might be on products they send overseas. Additionally, in-kind items (such as bleach and medical gloves) aren't as expensive for an entity to donate, so most organizations can find a way to give something.

Air transport

If medical workers become infected while in the affected areas and need to be evacuated out to their countries of residence, chartered flights can be very useful. Not many aircraft — at least in the United States — have the capacity to transport Ebola patients, but as the outbreak wears on, the need will probably increase.

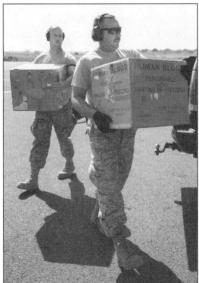

CDC Public Health Image Library

Figure 6-1: US Air National Guardsmen load blood donations from the Armed Services Blood Program for transport to Liberia.

Space

The International Charter on Space and Major Disasters provides for the charitable and humanitarian acquisition and transmission of space satellite data to relief organizations in the event of major disasters. Its images usually are used to make damage and hazard-assessment maps, but on October 9, the United States Geological Survey on behalf of the National Geospatial Agency activated it to monitor the outbreak in Sierra Leone, marking the first time its space assets have been used in an epidemiological role.

Education and outreach

To go beyond just stopping this outbreak and making sure that it doesn't happen again, education and outreach are essential. Agencies like UNICEF and Save the Children (more on them in Chapter 9) are coordinating and working with local community leaders to go into the cities and villages and educate the residents. However, these groups are definitely encountering some major challenges, mostly cultural in nature.

Many local residents don't believe that a virus causes Ebola; their belief system is more oriented toward blaming the sickness on black magic. Therefore, when someone comes to their home to give them supplies and teach them how to wash their hands with soap and water, they may not listen. Additionally, people in these areas are naturally skeptical of government and authorities, given their past with intense civil war and corruption, and won't even let western health officials be in their homes or villages. Hence, organizations must work in tandem with local anthropologists and residents. Community members themselves (and not outsiders) must talk to the residents.

Be careful of disrespecting or belittling West African beliefs. These beliefs are their religious and life-long value system, so to have westerners step on it, telling them how they should do things can be off-putting, offensive, and not effective at all.

Street teams made up of local residents who are advocates for their own families, friends, and communities are most effective at this work. Figures 6-2 and 6-3 show examples of messaging that's coming from within the community. One is in the form of an educational poster that's marked as being a message from the Liberian president, and the other is a homemade sign draped across a community leader's car. In Figure 6-4, a local community volunteer does outreach.

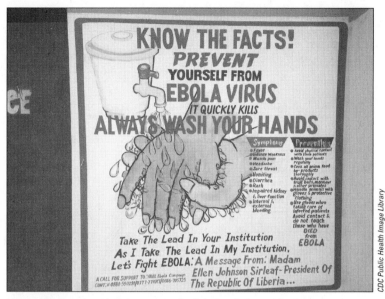

Figure 6-2: An educational message that's being delivered by the same community it's trying to reach is the most effective.

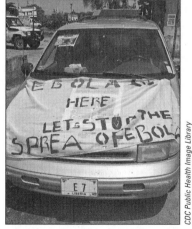

Figure 6-3: Educational messaging a cross the hood of a community leader's car in Liberia.

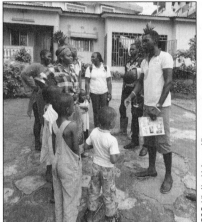

CDC Public Health Image Library

Figure 6-4: A volunteer with the Guinean Red Cross goes door-to-door to spread educational information about Ebola.

How the Outbreak Has Impacted the Area and World

The impact of this outbreak is starting to appear, and it will be awhile before the effect is fully realized in all the areas that it has affected or will affect. From agriculture to economy, travel to fighting other diseases, it's a wide-reaching event. These sections examine some of these areas.

Children

Ebola is leaving thousands (government officials estimate 26,000) of children — most under age 5 — without parents, without schools, and without a certain future. Not only are these children reeling from the death of their parents, they may be fighting Ebola themselves. Or if they have survived, they may be struggling against the stigmatism that so many survivors are feeling: Community members (sometimes even their own relatives) blame them for bringing Ebola into their villages and cities, and they are shunned. They have nowhere to go — not even school, because the schools have been closed in the wake of the outbreak.

Social workers, anthropologists, community leaders, and organizations like UNICEF and Save the Children (more on them in Chapter 9) are undertaking the effort to help kids connect with relatives who will house them, see to it that they make it to their new homes, launch emergency education sessions, and more to make sure these orphans don't fall through the cracks.

Churches are also playing a large role in caring for these orphans. During the outbreak, many doors are closed, but the churches remain open to the children.

Travel

Most countries have lifted wide bans on travel, but some countries are still sticking to them (*travel bans* basically are rules that prohibit people from certain countries from coming into others, regardless of health status; read more about them in Chapter 4). Keeping the bans in place causes big problems when trying to facilitate getting healthcare workers and supplies to and from the affected areas. One of these countries is the United Kingdom, which was supposed to lift a travel ban against flights from Sierra Leone on October 13, but then it decided to keep the ban, which drew protests from humanitarian organizations and airlines alike.

Meanwhile in the United States, a demonstration by Delta Airlines cabin cleaners at LaGuardia airport in New York City on October 9 and a press conference held by the National Nurses United (NNU) three days later, highlighted the need for basic safety information, training, and protective gear.

Agriculture

In Guinea, Liberia, and Sierra Leone, quarantine zones and restrictions on travel have seriously impacted the agriculture industry and food supply right in the middle of harvest season. The inability to harvest has led to massive food shortages. In turn, food prices have increased, in some cases, as much as 75 percent.

Outside of these countries, officials in the countries bordering the affected region are growing concerned about the impact that Ebola will have on their agriculture industry. Of particular note is cocoa. West Africa produces 70 percent of the world's global cocoa supply, and even though 60 percent of it is produced in Ghana and the Ivory Coast (which don't have outbreaks), those two countries are close enough to the affected area, that if the virus continues to spread, it could mean serious trouble there.

Economy

Several West African countries have significant numbers of foreign workers in critical sectors of the economy, and the fear of Ebola has caused almost a mass movement of them back to their home countries. In Ghana, for example, some global companies have evacuated non-essential foreign personnel (and Ghana doesn't even have any reported cases of Ebola).

For countries affected by the virus directly, it's much worse. Across Sierra Leone, Liberia, and Guinea, people are reluctant to stay there or come back after leaving, which includes the Chinese, who have invested heavily in Africa in recent years.

Overall, the World Bank estimates that the Liberian economy has declined by $113 million, Sierra Leone by $95 million, and Guinea by $120 million. It also warns that if the outbreak continues that the disease could cost the West African economy $32 billion in 2015.

The World Bank expects that GDP growth in Sierra Leone will only be 8.3 percent (down from 11.3 percent), with agriculture among the worst affected sectors; it also expects a slow in mining operations. Guinea's growth estimate is down more than 2 percent (from 4.5 to 2.4), and the worst hit sector is again agriculture. And Liberia, one of the smallest economies in the world, has had its growth projections reduced nearly 3.5 percent (from 5.9 to 2.5), with projections of zero or negative growth in 2015 — with mining and agriculture the worst hit sectors in the country.

Fear is powerful — and its reach can go much farther than you think. You might say, "So what if I don't want to go to West Africa right now? I'm only one person anyway." But if many people stop flying, change vacation plans, or cancel business contracts with this region, it quickly adds up. GDP growth rates will fall further, which impacts economies and markets around the world.

Trade

Trade within the affected area had been increasing thanks to government efforts. However, Ebola-related border closures by countries like Senegal, Ivory Coast, and Ghana — as well as travel bans — will have a significantly adverse effect on trade in the region.

Foreign investors are also postponing their investments. One of the things that makes West Africa so attractive for investment is the size of the market. The large number of sickness and deaths caused by Ebola has obviously impacted that benefit and will continue to do so.

Also, big projects are being halted. A World Bank contract for the construction of a road between Liberia and Guinea has been suspended because the Chinese contractor pulled out its workers.

Chapter 7

Just For Healthcare Workers: What You Need to Know

In This Chapter

▶ Taking care of your pre-trip exams and planning

▶ Using PPE and other protocols properly while in the affected areas

▶ Understanding travel screenings and restrictions

*A*s a healthcare worker who is currently on (or thinking about being on) the front lines in an affected area, you first should be thanked — so thank you! Secondly, I want to give you information that can help you prepare for and stay safe during your trip. And if you're still on the fence as to whether to go or not, I hope that I can help you make a decision. This chapter outlines what to do and expect before, during, and after your work in West Africa. Oh, and to those of you here who aren't healthcare workers, it's okay — you're welcome here to see what healthcare workers do to prepare to help save lives.

Planning before Your Trip

You have a lot to do before you leave. The better prepared you are, the more successful and safe your trip will be. Keep these pointers in mind before you depart:

✔ **Educate yourself.** Discover as much as you can about the virus in general, the current outbreak's history and progression, and the latest breaking news. Every day seems to have a new development, so staying on top of it all can be challenging. Make sure you know exactly what you're headed into.

✔ **Go to your own doctor four to six weeks before you leave.** Visit your travel medicine provider for an exam and updated vaccines. Discuss and develop a plan based on your medical history and travel needs.

- ✔ **Put together a travel health kit.** This kit should include prescription medicines, over-the-counter drugs, alcohol-based sanitizer, and a basic first aid kit.

- ✔ **Verify that your organization is providing you with PPE.** If it isn't giving you a personal protective equipment (PPE), then you should pack your own. Refer to the later section in this chapter, "Wearing the right gear: personal protective equipment (PPE)." (Flip to Chapter 4 for the items you need, or check the CDC website at www.cdc.gov.)

- ✔ **Take the CDC safety training course for healthcare workers going to West Africa.** The course is three days long and is offered most weeks in Atlanta. You can register online through www.cdc.train.org.

- ✔ **Make sure your health insurance covers illness abroad.** Ask your organization about medical evacuation plans (both if you have Ebola or if you have been exposed to it, but don't have symptoms). If you're not fully covered through your current health insurance and organization-provided evacuations, the CDC recommends that you purchase travel health insurance and medical evacuation insurance.

Some medical providers are excluding medical evacuation for people who have Ebola, so make sure you check carefully!

- ✔ **Know where you can receive medical care, should you need it, after you're there.** You may not have time to find out after you're there and if you really need it, so contact the US Embassy in your destination country ahead of time to inquire and then record the information.

- ✔ **Register with the US Embassy in your destination country.** You can do so through the US Department of State's Smart Traveler Enrollment Program (STEP) at www.step.state.gov.

Being Precautious during Your Trip

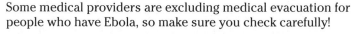

Even if you aren't in an area where Ebola patients are, this section is extremely important. And if you're in a high-risk area where people are infected with Ebola, this section is downright essential. That said, don't rely solely on this book as your only resource. Always attain and follow all guidance and training from your organization.

Wearing the right gear: personal protective equipment (PPE)

Your personal protective equipment (PPE) is your life preserver. If you don't put on the right gear, in the right order, and also take it off correctly, your risk of infection increases dramatically. You also put others at risk. Nothing is more important than your PPE. Chapter 4 outlines what the PPE for Ebola currently is.

Healthcare workers must follow detailed guidelines to follow when putting on and taking off PPEs, although the specifics are beyond the scope of this book. For these purposes, I outline the very basic rundown of donning here, just so you can get an idea:

1. **Engage the trained observer.**

2. **Remove your personal clothing and items.**

3. **Inspect your PPE prior to donning.**

4. **Perform hand hygiene.**

5. **Put on your inner gloves.**

6. **Put on your boots.**

7. **Put on your coveralls.**

8. **Put on your outer gloves.**

9. **Put on your respirator.**

10. **Put on your outer apron (if needed).**

11. **Verify.**

12. **Disinfect your outer gloves.**

After you have your PPE on, be really careful. Avoid touching or adjusting it yourself, changing gloves between patients, taking off damaged or torn gloves, and performing hand hygiene before putting on new gloves.

And here's the procedure for doffing (which should only be done in a designated PPE removal area):

1. **Engage trained observer.**

2. **Inspect.**

3. **Disinfect your outer gloves.**

4. **Remove your apron (if used).**

5. **Inspect.**

6. Disinfect your outer gloves.

7. Remove your boots.

8. Disinfect and remove your outer gloves.

9. Inspect and disinfect your inner gloves.

10. Remove your face shield.

11. Disinfect your inner gloves.

12. Remove your surgical hood.

13. Disinfect your inner gloves.

14. Remove your coveralls.

15. Disinfect and change your inner gloves.

16. Remove your respirator.

17. Disinfect your inner gloves.

18. Disinfect your washable shoes.

19. Disinfect and remove your inner gloves.

20. Perform hand hygiene.

21. Inspect.

22. You can wear scrubs outside of the PPE removal area.

23. Shower at the end of shift if you perform high-risk patient care.

24. Meet with infection specialist on site to evaluate care activities and assess any protocol concerns.

Identifying and isolating patients

Know the signs and symptoms of Ebola and develop a *triage system* (a process for prioritizing which patients to treat first) so Ebola patients can be identified and properly handled. Good screening procedures for identifying potential and actual patients are key. After you identify them, you should isolate them in a single room, if possible. If not, assign designated areas that are separate from other patients.

Within these designated areas, suspected and confirmed cases should also be separate. Also, the equipment used there should stay there. You should restrict access to these areas only to personnel who remain in service to only these areas. All other access should be prohibited, unless absolutely vital to the patients' well-being.

Preventing further infection

Although this section doesn't go into all of the technical and medical details, it gives you an overview of certain things that should always happen for infection prevention and control.

Wash your hands — Good hand hygiene

Hand hygiene is the most effective strategy for preventing the spread of infections in any healthcare setting, Ebola-affected settings included. You can use an alcohol-based hand sanitizer, soap and water, or in settings where neither is locally available, a mild (0.05 percent) chlorine solution.

You should perform hand hygiene in the following instances:

- ✔ Before you put on gloves and PPE on entry to an isolation room or area

- ✔ Before you perform any procedures on a patient

- ✔ After you've been in direct contact with a patient's body fluids or have been around a symptomatic patient

- ✔ After you touch anything that's been contaminated (or that you think is contaminated) in the patient's surroundings

- ✔ After you leave the isolation area and take off your PPE

If you don't perform hand hygiene after removing PPE, it will reduce the effectiveness of PPE. So *always* wash your hands!

Make sure that your facility has alcohol-based hand rubs at the entrances, exits, and within isolation wards and rooms. Although not needed at all points, make sure there's soap, running water, and disposable towels available somewhere nearby for all to access as well.

Disinfecting equipment and your environment

Other key precautions are safe injection and *phlebotomy* (blood draw) procedures, including safe management of sharps (such as not using devices that you need to disassemble after use and using puncture-resistant sharps containers), regular and rigorous environmental cleaning after patients leave room, and decontamination of surfaces and equipment with EPA-approved cleaning solution.

Identifying, isolating, and informing

Another major key to stopping the spread of Ebola is a standard for infection prevention that the CDC calls "Identify, isolate, and inform." You should perform this screening whenever a patient enters your facility. Refer to Chapter 4 for an overview.

Properly disposing of human remains

Human remains and medical waste associated with Ebola are highly contagious and must be handled according to specific and thorough guidelines. For the purposes of this book, I outline some parts of the major points as examples so you can get a sense of just how involved this process is. This little glimpse of a much larger process (and processes within processes) illustrates why the Ebola outbreak is so difficult to get under control. And keep in mind, too, that as conditions change, these protocols change. These guidelines are current as of the time of publishing.

General

The general principles for properly disposing of human remains apply to all of these situations:

- ✔ Unless you're trained in handling infected human remains and wearing PPE, you should not touch or move any Ebola-infected remains.

- ✔ In general, no one should handle human remains more than absolutely necessary.

- ✔ Don't perform autopsies on patients who die of Ebola. If you must perform one, consult the state health department and CDC regarding additional precautions.

- ✔ Always be respectful of patients' religious and cultural beliefs and requests. Accommodate as much as you can.

Safe and dignified burial

WHO has a very specific protocol for making sure that you preserve your own safety and the safety of the family and mourners during burials for Ebola victims. To review all 12 steps in detail, visit WHO's website at `www.who.int/csr/resources/publications/ebola/safe-burial-protocol/en/`.

Acting with the utmost sensitivity and compassion during the burial process is extremely important. Cultural differences, sudden and severe grief, and fear all bear down on the family, and it's your job to not add to their distress, but rather, lessen it as much as possible. Before you start anything, you must talk with and fully inform the family of the dignified burial process, which includes showing respect for the deceased. Also, as part of the informing step, give the family the formal agreement and only move forward with the process if the family agrees with it.

Postmortem preparation

At the site of death, wrap the body in a plastic shroud so that it can't contaminate the outside of it, then put the body in a leak-proof plastic bag and zip it closed. Then, put the body in another bag and zip it closed.

Decontaminate the surface of body bags by removing visible soil on outer bag. Then reapply the disinfectant to the entire bag surface and allow it to air dry. After the body has been removed, clean and disinfect the room, including any reusable equipment.

If your gown or gloves are heavily contaminated with blood or body fluids, change them. Don't remove IVs or endotracheal tubes. Don't wash or clean the body.

You don't have to wear PPE if you're only driving or riding in a vehicle carrying human remains, assuming that you've contained the remains properly, you don't handle them while transporting, and you disinfect the body bag.

Mortuary care

Here are some of the basic guidelines for mortuary care for Ebola patients:

- ✔ Don't perform embalming.

- ✔ Don't open body bags.

- ✔ Don't remove remains from body bags; just put them directly into a hermetically sealed casket.

- ✔ Wear PPE when handling bagged remains.

If any fluids leak from a bag, thoroughly clean and decontaminate areas with EPA-registered disinfectants, following label instructions. You should clean and disinfect reusable equipment according to standard procedures.

Disposing of remains

Here are some guidelines for disposition of remains:

- ✔ Cremate or bury remains right away in a hermetically sealed casket.

- ✔ After the body is bagged in a sealed casket, you don't have to do any additional cleaning, unless there is leakage.

- ✔ You don't need PPE to handle cremated remains or the hermetically sealed closed casket.

Transporting human remains

Here are some transportation guidelines:

✔ Keep transportation of remains to an absolute minimum.

✔ Coordinate all transport with relevant local and state authorities in advance.

✔ If you're transporting across state lines, coordinate with the CDC.

✔ If you need to transport remains to somewhere outside of the United States, you need to comply with the regulations of the country of destination, so coordinate with the proper officials ahead of time.

✔ If you properly incinerate, *autoclave* (steam-sterilize in a pressure chamber), or otherwise inactivate Ebola-infected material, it's no longer medical waste or hazardous material, so you can dispose of according to local regulations.

Knowing what to do if you get sick

If you get sick during your trip, first of all, act swiftly, but don't panic. Notify your organization that you have become ill. Make sure you know your point of contact and have that person's information with you at all times for this very reason (you may not be working together directly every day), and if you feel at all sick, don't second-guess it or wait. And if your organization instructs you to see a doctor or report to a specific medical facility, go directly there; don't make any stops anywhere else.

Taking Actions after Your Trip

After your service is complete (thank you again) and it's time to head home, you should expect to go through any number of screening procedures while traveling, and then possible monitoring, quarantining, or isolation once you're back in the states. These sections explain the procedures in greater depth.

Traveling on a jet plane

Well, you did it! You made it through your term of service and are ready to go back home. There are two processes to be prepared for: *exit screening* and *entry screening*. The exit screening is done at the airport of departure, whereas entry screening is done in the airport of your arrival.

Screening at the airport for either exit or entry can vary, but it'll probably look something like this:

✔ Get your temperature taken and be examined for signs and symptoms of illness. You'll also be asked to answer questions about your travel and potential exposure to Ebola. Be honest and fully participate.

✔ After the screening, authorities will decide if and when you can continue your trip.

✔ If you have symptoms of Ebola, you will not be allowed to travel commercially (it's also possible that even if you don't have symptoms, you may be denied travel still if you've been exposed to Ebola).

✔ If you have symptoms of Ebola, you may need to be medically evacuated to receive needed care.

✔ If you've been exposed to Ebola but aren't sick, you'll either have to arrange a charter flight home or stay in West Africa for at least 21 days until authorities ensure that it's safe for you to travel.

Here are some specifics about exit and entry screening:

Exit screening

People who have been exposed with Ebola or are sick with symptoms of Ebola won't be allowed to travel on commercial flights to the United States and potentially to other countries. The three international airports currently conducting exit screening are

✔ **Conakry** (Guinea)

✔ **Monrovia** (Liberia)

✔ **Freetown** (Sierra Leone)

Entry screening

You may need to be screened again when you arrive, depending on the country in which you land. Here is a partial list of current restrictions and airports doing *entry screening*:

✔ **United States:** Any passengers beginning their travels in Liberia, Sierra Leone, or Guinea can only enter the United States through the following airports: JFK International Airport, Newark International Airport, Dulles International Airport, Hartsfield-Jackson International Airport, O'Hare International Airport.

✔ **Canada:** Canada currently is not issuing visas to anyone who has recently visited the affected area in the past three months.

✔ **Australia:** Not issuing visas to anyone from Guinea, Liberia, and Sierra Leone, unless he holds permanent visas and has been quarantined for 21 days prior to arrival.

✔ **United Kingdom:** People arriving from Sierra Leone, Liberia, or Guinea to London Heathrow, London Gatwick, Birmingham, or Manchester airports are screened about travel and exposure history. They may be subject to a medical assessment given by medical professionals. Screening is also happening at London St. Pancras station for Eurostar.

Remember, this is only current as of time of publication, so you should always double check with the CDC, WHO, and local jurisdictions for most updated information.

Returning to your humble abode

Assuming you aren't under quarantine or in isolation (refer to Chapter 4 for more about quarantines and isolation), you'll need to do a few other things, including the following:

✔ **If you were exposed to Ebola during your trip, call your doctor and local health department even if you don't have symptoms.** Your doctor should evaluate your exposure level and symptoms if you have them and consult with public health authorities to determine whether actions, such as medical evaluation and testing for Ebola, monitoring, or travel restrictions are needed.

✔ **Monitor your health for 21 days if you were in an area with an Ebola outbreak.** During the time that you're monitoring your health, you can continue your normal activities, including work.

✔ **Even if you weren't exposed to Ebola, you should still pay attention to your health after you return.** Although you should know if you were exposed, it's possible you may not, so be extra cognizant of how you feel.

✔ **Watch for other Ebola symptoms.** They can include severe headache, muscle pain, vomiting, diarrhea, stomach pain, or unexplained bleeding or bruising. Refer to Chapter 5 for more information about symptoms.

✔ **Take your temperature every morning and evening.** Normal temperature is 98.6 degrees F (37 degrees C). If yours is above that slightly, be sure to note it for yourself and watch it.

If your temperature is 100.4 degrees F (38 degrees C) or higher or you have any other Ebola symptoms, separate yourself from others, notify the local health department, seek medical care immediately, and follow the other guidance in the earlier "Knowing what to do if you get sick" section.

Part IV

The Part of Tens

Go to www.dummies.com/extras/ebolamythsandfacts for a list of ten ways that you can't contract Ebola.

In this part . . .

- ✔ Discover how far off a vaccine for Ebola is from being available and what a vaccine can do to prevent the disease from spreading.

- ✔ Comprehend why contracting Ebola doesn't have to be a death sentence.

- ✔ See what other diseases and health conditions, including antibiotic resistance, are significant and could be significant health crises.

Chapter 8

Ten Myths Clearly Busted about Ebola

● ●

In This Chapter

▶ Uncovering whether there's a cure

▶ Isolating people with symptoms

▶ Knowing how to kill the virus

● ●

*O*ver the course of the 2014 Ebola outbreak, a lot of media coverage, online banter, all kinds of analysis, and water cooler chatter have been running rampant. With so much information (and opinion) flying in all directions, you can easily get swept up in misinformation — not to mention, new cases pop up, old cases have developments, and scientists are making more discoveries every day. With such a large body of information in your face every day, you can start to feel at least a little uneasy.

So what should you believe and what should you dismiss? What's fact, what are guesses, and what are downright myths? Figuring it out is sometimes difficult, but it's important that you do. The more you know about Ebola, the less you will fear (and the more you can share with others). Throughout this book I provide lots of facts that debunk the common myths about Ebola. This chapter zeros in on some of the most common myths about Ebola and busts them in one easy location.

Ebola Is Highly Contagious

Although Ebola is highly *infectious* (meaning that it doesn't take much of the virus to infect someone), it isn't very *contagious* (capable of being transmitted from one person to another) — especially in the United States, Canada, and Western Europe. It's actually rather difficult to catch Ebola.

Why? Infected body fluids have to come in direct contact with your mucus membranes or a skin opening (refer to Chapter 4 for more information on transmission).

Ebola isn't airborne, which means that if an infected patient sneezes large droplets of body fluid into the air, the virus doesn't just stay there, like say, chickenpox germs do.

In order to actually infect you, the droplets have to actually land on your mucus membranes or non-intact skin. Although the virus *can* live for a short time on a surface, it soon dies as the droplet around it evaporates.

Ebola Has a Cure and a Vaccine

Ebola has neither a cure nor a vaccine — at least not yet. Scientists are fast-tracking their research and development, and it looks promising. Some say experimental vaccines could be shipped to West Africa as early as January or February of 2015; look at Chapter 5 for details.

Progress also is being made on the treatment and cure front; however, its fate is a little less clear. The experimental drug, ZMapp, created by Mapp Biopharmaceutical, has been given to a small handful of patients (all non-West Africans), and most of them survived. The problem is that the pharmaceutical company is out of the drug, and it's unknown when more will be available.

The whole issue of using drugs and medicines during this outbreak is tricky because all are experimental at this juncture, which means they haven't been tested on humans, so researchers don't know a whole lot about the side effects.

All drugs, before the Food and Drug Administration (FDA) approves them for usage in the United States, must go through randomized clinical trials. A *randomized clinical trial* is an experiment in which the people in the study are randomly assigned to one of the treatment groups — without knowing which one they're assigned to. All subjects then follow the same protocols and undergo the same testing so the treatments can be compared and assessed without bias.

Clinical trials are necessary to prove the effectiveness of a new medication. Unless such trials are done — which is very difficult in a resource-poor setting in the midst of a public health emergency — being able to prove that a patient's recovery was due to a specific medication is impossible.

Ebola Is a Death Sentence

Ebola isn't necessarily a death sentence. In West Africa, surviving Ebola is less likely, because West African countries don't have any of the needed health infrastructure (such as enough doctors — before the outbreak, Liberia had one doctor for every 100,000 people) that could've addressed the outbreak before it reached the current level, or treat it fully now that it's in full swing.

As long as you identify and report symptoms immediately and get medical care early, your chances of survival are better. People who have Ebola need urgent hospitalization in order to survive because — among other things — they need the following:

- ✔ **IV fluids:** Because patients are losing so much fluid, they're at high risk for dehydration. The IVs keep them hydrated at the proper levels to support organ function.

- ✔ **Pain medication:** Ebola patients suffer from muscle and joint pain. Alleviating this pain with medication can help keep the patients comfortable.

- ✔ **Monitoring of organ function:** The Ebola virus attacks the immune system and causes the blood pressure to fall, which in turn compromises various organs because they don't get enough blood, which carries oxygen. Patients must be monitored constantly to prevent organ failure.

- ✔ **Intensive nursing:** Ebola patients' conditions can change very rapidly, and they require frequent monitoring of temperature, pulse, blood pressure, respiratory status, level of consciousness, and intake and output of fluids. On top of that, patients often need regular linen changes and cleanups.

Many people who get treated outside of West Africa make full recoveries from Ebola. However, in West Africa, not all locals believe in western medicine, doctors, or hospital settings. Many villagers prefer using healers or medicine men, so they may not access the medical care they need in time. Also, they watch others get taken to medical centers to receive care when they're extremely ill, and when those folks end up dying, the remaining villagers draw a faulty conclusion that the doctors are the ones who killed them. For more on treating Ebola, turn to Chapter 5.

Anyone Who Has Ebola Symptoms Should Be Isolated

Isolating (separating a person in a special medical room or ward for the duration of treatment) anyone who has Ebola symptoms (flip to Chapter 5 to see the symptoms) is a severe overreaction that would lead to unnecessary resource drain and public hysteria. Ebola symptoms are so common in the early stages (they're pretty much exactly like flu symptoms), that officials would end up needing to isolate much of the country this flu season, only to discover that it's not Ebola.

The only people who need to be isolated are those who are showing Ebola-like symptoms *and* who have been exposed to outbreak areas or confirmed Ebola patients.

You're probably more familiar with the term *quarantine* (which is a 21-day period of confinement to make sure someone doesn't have Ebola) because it's on the news a lot. A quarantine happens to people who have been exposed to outbreak areas or confirmed Ebola patients but *don't* have symptoms themselves.

The United States Isn't Ready

West Africa wasn't ready for Ebola, but the United States is. The US healthcare leaders have learned from and evolved through this country's past experiences with health emergencies, such as pandemic flu and SARS. The government and healthcare leaders have built a sophisticated and thorough infrastructure of policies, protocols, and facilities over time.

And now, with this Ebola outbreak, healthcare professionals have taken the opportunity to prepare hospitals with the right space, equipment, and additional training specific to Ebola, should they need it.

Additionally, the United States has a good system in place for *contact tracing,* which enables healthcare providers to quickly identify and monitor possible Ebola patients before they become symptomatic.

So at the end of the day, this country is indeed ready — probably more than needed. In fact, you might say that it's all dressed up with no place to go. But that's much better than the alternative, as the folks in the affected areas are all too well aware of.

Ebola Is the World's Biggest Public Health Threat

Although Ebola currently is one of the biggest public health threats in West Africa, overall it's not the biggest public health threat for the world. Ebola is considered a fairly rare disease and outbreaks aren't often seen — and certainly not to this extent.

US leaders can't make the mistake of paying so much attention to Ebola — the unlikely killer in the United States, Canada, and Western Europe that it is — that they ease up on prevention, education, and monitoring of more likely threats (read about those threats in Chapter 10). Case in point: One of the terrible impacts of the Ebola outbreak is that it has caused West Africa's progress in the fight against malaria to backslide (to find out how else the Ebola outbreak has impacted the world, turn to Chapter 6).

You Need a Special Substance to Kill the Ebola Virus

Amazingly enough, Ebola is just like any other virus: You can kill it by washing your hands with soap and water. Hand hygiene is a key piece to prevention and treatment in the outbreak areas. An alcohol-based hand sanitizer can also work (as long as the hands aren't actually visibly soiled). Just like your mother taught you: Wash your hands with soap and water regularly to stay healthy.

For disinfecting Ebola isolation areas, bleach-based environmental cleaning supplies are often used, and all hospital-grade disinfectants are effective. Chapter 4 has more on prevention.

Bringing Ebola Patients to the United States Puts You at Risk

Having Ebola patients brought to the United States for treatment doesn't put you or other Americans at risk for an outbreak. The difficulty of contracting the virus, combined with the infrastructure, makes the risks extremely low.

In fact, some argue that the United States should bring more patients here for treatment, where the healthcare system has the capacity, equipment, and staff to successfully care for them.

Ebola Liquefies Your Organs, Which Causes the Bleeding

This myth is a perfect example of slight truths being twisted and re-invented. Ebola doesn't liquefy your organs. In a minority of cases, hemorrhaging from the eyes, mouth, ears, and nose does happen, but it's because Ebola weakens the blood vessels and prevents the blood from clotting. What usually ultimately causes death is multi-organ failure and shock. Chapter 2 has more on what the virus does to your body.

This Current Outbreak Is Unusually Strong and Deadly

This strain of Ebola has been around since its discovery in 1976. It hasn't changed or mutated; the reason this outbreak is so much worse than all the other ones throughout history comes down to several reasons:

✔ West Africa has never had an outbreak of this magnitude, so health officials weren't on the lookout for it and didn't recognize the danger as fast as they could have.

✔ It started in an area that has particularly porous borders. That is, people move back and forth freely and often over the borders in that region for work, farming, markets, and so forth. That meant the virus was already in three countries before anyone realized it.

✔ As compared to many of the previous outbreaks that happened in remote villages, this one reached urban centers early, and the density helped the virus spread very fast.

✔ West African death rituals involve a lot of touching and washing of bodies, so many people regularly came (and still come) into contact with infected body fluids without realizing it. (Refer to Chapter 4 for more information about how death rituals can transmit the virus.)

✔ Guinea, Sierra Leone, and Liberia are three of the poorest countries in the world. They don't have the infrastructure or medical care to address Ebola. As an illustration, these three countries have a patient-doctor ratio of around 100,000 to 1. (Check out Chapter 3 for more about the countries in West Africa that have been most affected.)

Chapter 9

Ten Organizations That Are Helping Fight Ebola

In This Chapter

▶ Donating to reputable organizations

▶ Finding out where you can volunteer

▶ Supporting the people who support the patients

*W*henever serious tragedies occur around the world, people and organizations from all corners of the globe always respond to the need for help, whether it be with funds, supplies, or manpower. It's also a time that unfortunately brings out scam artists and opportunists. Often, people want to help by donating something or even volunteering, but knowing who to trust or which organizations are providing services that are most needed can be difficult.

With an international event, such as the Ebola outbreak of 2014, transparency can be a challenge. Consider this example: If a large tornado destroyed several houses and businesses in your hometown and everyone pitched in to help rebuild and assist affected families, the results would be right in front of you. You'd be able to give help directly to those in need. But with a situation like an Ebola outbreak in West Africa, providing direct help is difficult, if not impossible. Donors have to rely on nonprofit organizations to provide the help.

In this chapter, I present ten trusted organizations that are helping in West Africa in various ways. I also include a few personal stories and updates from people who benefit from the work these organizations do.

 If you're still wary, you can always check out the organization on Charity Navigator, which is a nonprofit run by the IRS to review all charities in the United States. Go to www.charitynavigator. org for more information.

You can find a list of points to consider when figuring out which charity you may want to consider at www.dummies.com/extras/ebolamythsandfacts.

Partners in Health

Partners In Health (PIH) (www.pih.org) is based in Boston, Massachusetts, and supports two grassroots organizations: Last Mile Health in Liberia and Wellbody Alliance in Sierra Leone. The organization trains health workers, strengthens medical clinics, and expands medical services beyond the urban centers. It also has formed rapid response teams to investigate remote areas where clusters of Ebola cases have appeared, and then execute care for sick patients, and education for the community.

Its mission is "to provide a preferential option for the poor in healthcare. By establishing long-term relationships with sister organizations based in settings of poverty, Partners In Health strives to achieve two overarching goals: to bring the benefits of modern medical science to those most in need of them and to serve as an antidote to despair."

Save the Children

Thanks in part to a large grant from philanthropist Paul G. Allen, Save the Children (www.savethechildren.org) is focusing its efforts on the (according to UNICEF) 3,700 children who are orphaned because of Ebola. The organization works primarily in Liberia to trace relatives of the children and arrange for re-homing. It also provides follow-up psychosocial services to make sure the child and family are doing well. Survivors of Ebola (and relatives of the dead) are often stigmatized by the community. Save the Children's work combats that through programming and support that addresses violence and abuse.

Save the Children also is working to provide emergency education programs (including education by radio) in light of the local schools being shuttered from the epidemic.

Save the Children's mission is to "invest in childhood — every day, in times of crisis and for the future. In the United States and around the world, the organization gives children a healthy start, the opportunity to learn, and protection from harm."

Doctors Without Borders/Medecins Sans Frontieres (MSF)

Doctors Without Borders (www.doctorswithoutborders.org) is the main organization providing medical care on the ground in West Africa. The organization has responded to more than 12 Ebola outbreaks since 1995. Doctors Without Borders began responding to the current West African outbreak in March 2014, where it has more than 3,000 people deployed to help the affected regions.

The organization operates six Ebola case management centers in West Africa and has cared for about 3,200 confirmed Ebola patients, in addition to caring for thousands of others who are sick. Additionally, it has shipped more than 1,019 tons of supplies to the affected countries since March.

MSF was founded in 1971, and its mission is "to help people worldwide where the need is the greatest, delivering emergency medical aid to people affected by conflict, epidemics, disasters, or exclusion from healthcare."

CDC Foundation

The CDC Foundation (www.cdcfoundation.com), which is the nonprofit arm of the Centers for Disease Control and Prevention, has deployed 160 staff members and 700 support staff to West Africa since July 2014.

Recently, the foundation received a $25 million donation from Facebook CEO Mark Zuckerberg and his wife Dr. Priscilla Chan. The money has enabled the foundation to continue to build and manage an emergency operations center, which is essential to the success of the outbreak response. Within these operations, it collects and monitors data to identify cases early, designs and enforces protocols for responding to cases, and coordinates various partner organizations on the ground.

The foundation also provides supplies and equipment, such as infection control tools, ready-to-eat meals, generators, vehicles, and supplies at airports (for instance, thermal scanners to detect fever). Its mission is "to help the CDC do more, faster by forging effective partnerships between CDC and safety."

International Federation of Red Cross and Red Crescent Societies

The International Red Cross and Red Crescent Movement (IFRC) (www.ifrc.org) is the world's largest humanitarian network, composed of almost 100 million members, volunteers, and supporters in 189 national societies. It provides five kinds of protection and assistance to people affected by disasters and conflicts in a totally neutral way (free of politics or religion): disaster relief, support for military families, blood supplies, health and safety services, and international services.

The IFRC has more than 7,700 volunteers and 170 Red Cross delegates in affected regions in West Africa, and the organization's work will reach 39 million people. The Red Cross opened the first treatment clinic in Sierra Leone; it manages 100 percent of the burials in Guinea; and it trains health workers in disinfecting equipment, disposing of waste, and increasing public awareness, among many other tasks.

Americares

Americares (www.americares.org) supports the frontline healthcare workers through shipments of supplies. So far, it has shipped more than 3.6 million items of safety and treatment supplies, including 2.6 million units of protective gear and other supplies.

In addition, Americares helps map out containment strategies in Sierra Leone and Liberia. The organization needs support in the form of donations and volunteers, if you're a healthcare professional.

Americares is a nonprofit emergency response and global health organization, whose mission is: "In times of epic disaster or daily struggle, we deliver medical and humanitarian aid to people in need worldwide."

CARE

CARE (www.care.org) is working with community leaders to educate people about the signs of Ebola, how to report potential cases, where to go for treatment, and proper hygiene. CARE also distributes household hand-washing stations that include buckets, chlorine water, soap, gloves, and educational posters about Ebola prevention.

CARE is a leading humanitarian organization fighting global poverty. Through community-based efforts focused on empowering women, the organization prevents the spread of disease, increases access to clean water and sanitation, expands economic opportunity, and protects natural resources. CARE also delivers emergency aid to survivors of war and natural disasters.

UNICEF

UNICEF's (www.unicef.org) focus is to support communities to protect themselves and to be able to access basic healthcare if any of their members contract Ebola. In Sierra Leone, UNICEF and partners have visited around 80 percent of all households in the country to give them educational material on Ebola and find any sick people.

The organization also has opened ten basic health facilities in rural parts of Sierra Leone, which makes early identification and access to healthcare more possible, which is vital in treatment, recovery, and prevention. UNICEF is also the largest supplier of the equipment for the response, including personal protective equipment (PPE). (Refer to Chapter 4 for more about PPE.)

UNICEF is also working to help children and young people who have been affected by Ebola in West Africa, and has sent emergency medical supplies to affected regions. The organization also worked to provide public education. One of its more unique programs is the outreach that it's doing for visually impaired people. Together with the Sierra Leonean government, UNICEF has helped to develop Ebola messaging in Braille.

Part of the group's mission is "to respond in emergencies to protect the rights of children. In coordination with United Nations partners and humanitarian agencies, UNICEF makes its unique facilities for rapid response available to its partners to relieve the suffering of children and those who provide their care."

Emergency USA

Emergency USA (www.emergencyusa.org) "helps bring lifesaving care to war-torn communities around the globe through sustainable regional medical centers that provide healthcare services to men, women, and children free of charge."

The organization has built the first and only fully functioning treatment center in Sierra Leone, and is currently trying to raise money to fund a larger 90-bed facility in the same location. Donations being raised now go to this initiative, as well as helping get medical supplies and materials to the treatment center's staff of 200.

GlobalGiving's Ebola Relief Fund

GlobalGiving (www.globalgiving.org/ebola/) is "an online marketplace that connects you to the causes and countries you care about." Within this marketplace, you select the projects you want to support, make a donation, and get regular progress reports.

Currently, it has an Ebola Relief Fund that is quite extensive, beyond just the $1 million it has raised. Within the fund (and you see this on its website), GlobalGiving has all kinds of projects that the group is funneling funds to for the Ebola outbreak. The money goes to various kinds of local aid organizations and funds medical supplies, protective equipment, and educational campaigns.

What's really interesting is that you can select which particular program or group you want your money to go to, and then later, you get updates from the field about how the program is doing.

Chapter 10

Ten Global Health Threats in Addition to Ebola

***

In This Chapter

▶ Comprehending why overuse of antibiotics is a problem

▶ Understanding why measles could make a comeback in the United States

▶ Remembering that HIV is still a problem

***

*W*hile the world is focused on West Africa as it experiences the worst Ebola outbreak in history and fears of a worldwide Ebola epidemic ensue, thousands of other diseases wage their wars against public health, too. The irony is that when you compare Ebola to other global health threats you see that it's not the worst-case scenario. The world's fight against Ebola is valid, but society has to be careful not to lose sight of the big picture that includes other threats, such as the ones that I discuss in this chapter.

Influenza

Every year, influenza kills about 36,000 and hospitalizes 200,000 more in the United States alone. During the 2013–2014 flu season, more than 100 children died from the flu. In fact, the flu ranks number seven on the CDC's list of ten top killers.

Most people think flu is only dangerous for elderly folks or young children, but the 2013–2014 flu season was especially bad for young adults. The irony is that a vaccine is available for influenza, but only a third of Americans get their annual flu shots.

Additionally, pneumonia can sometimes develop along with or right after someone gets the flu, which is even deadlier. The concurrence happens because a lot of (even healthy) people carry bacteria that can cause pneumonia in their noses. Because there's so much mucus and sneezing and blowing involved with the flu, that bacteria can end up in the lungs, which is where it turns into pneumonia.

Here's how you can protect yourself from influenza:

- ✔ **If you're older than six months of age (and obviously you are because you're reading this book), then you should get a flu vaccine.** Several different flu vaccines are available. They all protect against the most common types of flu, and some have different delivery methods. (For example, one shot goes under your skin instead of your muscle, and another vaccine is a nasal spray.) Talk to your doctor or pharmacist to find out which one is right for you.

- ✔ **Cough and sneeze into the crook of your elbow or a tissue.** Covering your cough or sneeze this way can prevent any viruses that you might be carrying from being sent into the air where they can infect others. Don't use your hands to cover your mouth or nose. Using your hands makes it more likely that you'll transfer the virus directly (with a handshake) or indirectly (by touching an object that someone else then touches) to someone else.

- ✔ **Wash your hands frequently.** Soap and water and alcohol-based hand cleansers are highly effective at killing most viruses and germs. Get in the habit of washing them regularly to keep yourself from spreading germs.

- ✔ **If you're sick, stay home from work or school.** Sometimes, people think toughing it out and showing up to work (or school) sick is the right thing to do. It's like they think, "Hey, look how committed and responsible I am. Even though I don't feel so hot, I'm still going to do my job." That's great and all until you infect the whole office. Just do everyone a favor and keep yourself (and germs) at home.

Antibiotic Resistance

More than 2 million people in the United States develop an infection from antibiotic-resistant bacteria annually. The CDC estimates that at least 23,000 people die from those infections each year.

Infections and diseases that were once cured by a safe, inexpensive, and simple medication now require broader spectrum (cover many different types of bacteria), less safe, and more expensive antibiotics to treat. There have been increases in antibiotic-resistant staph infections, gonorrhea, and something called carbapenem resistant enterobacteriaceae (CRE), which are resistant to most available antibiotics, among others, which means long and painful and (pricey) hospitalizations while doctors find a way to kill the superbugs.

Methicillin-resistant Staphylococcus aureus, or *MRSA,* is one of the most prevalent infections. According to the CDC, about 80,000 people are diagnosed with MRSA each year and 11,000 people die. MRSA can be spread through skin-to-skin contact and contact with infected materials, such as surgical tools or breathing tubes. It's a problem in healthcare facilities and now commonly occurs in the community.

Here is how you can protect yourself against antibiotic resistance:

- ✔ **Wash your hands with warm water and soap or properly sanitize the hands with alcohol-based cleansers.**

- ✔ **Appropriately use antibiotics.** Don't use them very much, and use them only when absolutely necessary.

- ✔ **Choose foods that are raised organically and without antibiotics.** Because antibiotics are so rampant in the factory farming industry, you can pretty much bet that you consume antibiotics every day. When making your food choices, select antibiotic-free produce and meats as much as possible. If you can, use farmers' markets, where you can talk with the actual farmers to discover more about how your food is raised.

Measles

In 2013, WHO reported that there were 145,700 measles deaths worldwide. Measles cases in the United States skyrocketed in 2014 (about 600 cases were reported from January to August alone, compared to less than 200 in *all* of 2013, and less than 100 in 2012). This rapid and large increase is a huge problem. One in every thousand children who contract measles will die, and all of them get extremely ill. (Some actually go deaf or suffer from permanent brain damage.)

The reason for this increase: Too many parents have chosen to stop vaccinating their children altogether, causing massive outbreaks. In fact, some cities in the United States have vaccination rates lower than that of a developing country. Babies of unvaccinated mothers are at the greatest risk. They're too young for the vaccine and lack immunity from their mothers. Of the estimated 600 measles cases in 2014, nearly all were in children.

Many parents have chosen not to vaccinate due to fears that vaccines can cause autism. A study from the United Kingdom often cited by the antivaccine movement comes from Dr. Andrew Wakefield, which suggested that there was a link between the measles-mumps-rubella (MMR) vaccine and autism. The British General Medical Council found his study to be fraudulent and his license was revoked, but not before it fed antivaccine fears that are now often perpetuated by celebrities who have no science or medical background.

To protect yourself against measles is simple: For best protection, the CDC recommends vaccinating your children twice: once when they are 12 to 15 months old, and again when they are 4 to 6 years old. If you've already been vaccinated, then you don't have anything to worry about. People who have had the measles, and those born before January 1, 1957 are also considered to be immune and don't require vaccination.

Drug-Resistant Tuberculosis

According to WHO, there are 500,000 new cases of drug-resistant tuberculosis per year worldwide. The treatment is long and hard, and fraught with side effects. Tuberculosis kills the second-highest amount of people among illnesses that contain only one pathogen (behind HIV/AIDS).

Drug resistance arises when the course of antibiotics is interrupted and the levels of drug in the body can't kill all of the bacteria.

This interruption can happen for a number of reasons:

- ✔ When patients start feeling better, they sometimes stop taking their medications (when they should finish the course).
- ✔ Drug supplies may not be available in the quantities needed (or at all) in parts of the world where TB is more common.
- ✔ Patients can forget to take their medication (or get lazy).
- ✔ Patients don't receive proper treatment.

Here is how drug-resistant TB can be prevented by physicians and patients:

- ✔ **Quickly diagnose TB cases.** The sooner TB is discovered, the better the chances are for not developing resistance.
- ✔ **Follow recommended treatment guidelines.** If the proper dosing and duration isn't given, resistance can develop.
- ✔ **Monitor patients' response to treatment.** Look for symptoms, which commonly include fever, chills, cough, night sweats, and weight loss, improving with treatment.

> ✔ **Make sure therapy is completed.** Stopping treatment before the full course is finished makes the patient susceptible to resistance.

Congenital Syphilis

This type of syphilis occurs when a mother passes on the disease to her unborn child in utero. Congenital syphilis is a neglected health problem, and many countries don't invest in the cost-effective prevention, diagnosis, and treatment measures to stop it.

The fetus is at greatest risk of contracting syphilis when the mother is in the early stages of both the illness and her pregnancy, but the disease can be passed at any stage of pregnancy, even during delivery. If a pregnant mother receives treatment (especially before week 16), the chances are very good that the fetus won't contract syphilis. If the mother is in the secondary stage of syphilis, getting treatment before the last month of pregnancy decreases the risk of transmission to the baby by 98 percent.

If the child does contract it, he can be treated with antibiotics much like an adult, but any developmental damage can't be reversed.

Malaria

In 2012 alone, malaria killed somewhere in the range of 627,000 people worldwide. The people living in the poorest countries (pretty much right where the Ebola outbreak is) are most vulnerable to it. Before Ebola struck, these countries were waging a promising battle against malaria, but the current Ebola outbreak has taken away all resources that they had for it, so in fact, even more people are dying of malaria right now.

Malaria is a serious and sometimes fatal disease caused by a parasite that may be carried by a certain type of mosquito that feeds on humans. In other words, it's not contagious; people can't give it directly to one another. Symptoms of malaria include high fevers, shaking chills, and flulike illness.

There is effective treatment, but prevention is far better than treating a serious disease. If you're going to be going to an area that has malaria, you should visit your doctor to acquire anti-malarial pills, which are taken throughout the trip and for one to four weeks after return. Also, be sure to use a mosquito net, wear clothes that cover your skin, and spray yourself with mosquito repellent. The best protection is obtained with a DEET-containing repellent on exposed skin and one that contains permethrin sprayed on outer clothing.

Helminths

Helminths are intestinal worms (roundworms, whipworms, and hookworms) that are transmitted through soil. The WHO estimates that more than one billion people have them. Because they're transmitted through fecal matter that ends up in the ground soil, helminths are more prevalent in areas that don't have well-developed hygiene and sanitation systems, but they can occur in the United States and Canada.

They can't be transmitted directly from person to person, or even from fresh feces, because eggs need about three weeks to mature in the soil before they become infective.

Typically, people residing in at-risk areas are periodically treated with de-worming medication regardless of diagnosis. The medication is given once a year when the prevalence of soil-transmitted helminth infections in the community is more than 20 percent and twice a year when the prevalence of soil-transmitted helminth infections in the community is more than 50 percent. Also, community education and outreach tries to promote good hygiene.

HIV/AIDS

More than 35 million people in the world have HIV. In the United States, that number is more than a million, and one in every six of those infected don't know that they are infected, so they spread it unknowingly. After the brutality and ignorance of the 1980s and early 1990s, the progress in the 2000s has been great, but it's lulled many people into thinking that HIV/AIDS isn't a problem anymore. People aren't dying from AIDS immediately like they used to; they're living for decades now if they have access to the current medications. As a result, HIV/AIDS has fallen off the radar for a lot of folks, but it's still a global health problem.

It targets the immune system and weakens a person's ability to fight infections and some types of cancer. As the virus destroys and impairs the function of immune cells, infected individuals gradually become immunodeficient.

HIV is transmitted through body fluids from infected individuals, such as blood, breast milk, semen, and vaginal secretions.

You can reduce the risk of contracting HIV by doing the following:

- ✔ **If you choose to have sex, use condoms all the time, even if it's with a regular sex partner.** All it takes is once without protection for the virus to spread, so use one every time you have sex.

- ✔ **Get tested regularly.** You should get tested for HIV every year. (You can do it during your annual checkup.) If you're engaged in high-risk activities (such as needle sharing or unprotected sex), you should get tested every three to six months. Early detection often means better treatment results.

- ✔ **If you inject drugs, access harm-reduction-based needle exchanges.** IV drug use puts you at severe risk for HIV, so you shouldn't do it at all. But if you do, find a source for clean needles, and don't share needles with anyone.

- ✔ **Consider taking newly released PrEP.** PrEP is pre-exposure prophylaxis that you take every day if you feel you are at risk for contracting HIV. Studies have shown PrEP results in a 92 percent reduction in risk.

Polio

Franklin D. Roosevelt contracted polio in 1921, before he was elected President of the United States. He did great work to advance the study of polio before even taking office. One of his contributions was the founding of a hydrotherapy center for polio patients. He found that water therapy was helpful for him, so he opened a center in Georgia in 1926, which still operates to this day. Additionally, FDR helped found the March of Dimes, a foundation that supports the rehabilitation of polio patients and supported the work of Jonas Salk, which ultimately led to a polio vaccine. This, in turn, led to eradication of polio in the United States by 1979.

Fast-forward to today. Polio was on its way to being eradicated worldwide, but 2014 has seen an unprecedented spread of it to new countries. The resurgence was caused by the Taliban prohibiting vaccinations in Pakistan and so it spread to Afghanistan. It has spread from Syria to Iraq as a result of people fleeing from civil unrest, and from Cameroon to Equatorial Guinea. Unlike Ebola, you can spread polio even if you don't have symptoms, so vaccinating against it is key to stopping an outbreak. Although no cases have been reported in the United States for decades, with the current trend, where some parents don't vaccinate their children, there is a chance it will re-emerge here, too.

Polio is an infectious disease caused by a virus. It invades the nervous system and can cause irreversible paralysis in a matter of hours — and it can be transmitted from person to person.

The virus enters the body through the mouth and multiplies in the intestine. It is then shed into the environment through the feces, and if it's in a country with poor sanitation, it can spread fast. However, if a sufficient number of children are fully immunized against polio, the virus is unable to find susceptible children to infect and dies out. So the vaccine is truly the key to stopping this disease.

What's really scary and dangerous is that people may have no signs of illness and are never aware they have been infected. They can carry the virus in their intestines and spread the infection to thousands of others before the first case of paralytic polio emerges. For this reason, WHO considers a single confirmed case of paralytic polio to be evidence of an epidemic — particularly in countries where very few cases occur.

Chagas Disease

This disease is transmitted through the feces of triatomine bugs that live in the cracks of poorly constructed homes in rural or suburban areas, and it affects 7 to 8 million people worldwide. It used to be limited just to Latin America, but has since been reported in the United States, Canada, and Europe. The cost of treatment for Chagas disease remains substantial. In Colombia alone, the annual cost of medical care for all patients with the disease was estimated to be about $267 million in 2008.

Symptoms include difficulty breathing, abdominal pain, and even death in later stages. Although it can be treated, there is no vaccine, so *vector control* (eliminating the creatures that are responsible for spreading disease) is a key measure in prevention. Early treatment is essential for those infected, because the cardiac disease that occurs in later stages can't be cured. Great progress has been made in vector management since the 1990s in Latin America.

To prevent yourself from getting Chagas disease:

✔ Sleep indoors in well-constructed buildings.

✔ Use bed nets treated with insecticides.

✔ Wear protective clothing.

✔ Apply insect repellent to exposed skin.

About the Author

Edward Chapnick, MD, is Director of the Division of Infectious Diseases and Vice Chairman of Medicine at Maimonides Medical Center in Brooklyn, New York. His practice includes the treatment of patients with a wide range of problems in the specialty of infectious diseases, including HIV, antibiotic-resistant bacterial infections, and travel medicine.

He received his MD degree from the State University of New York, Downstate Medical Center, and completed his training in Internal Medicine and Infectious Diseases at the Maimonides Medical Center. He is a fellow of the American College of Physicians, the Infectious Diseases Society of America, and the Society for Healthcare Epidemiology of America. His activities also include teaching, and he is a professor of clinical medicine at the Albert Einstein College of Medicine in the Bronx, New York. Dr. Chapnick has numerous publications in the peer-reviewed medical literature and is actively engaged in clinical research.

Dedication

This book is dedicated to the patients and families who have experienced the devastation of the Ebola epidemic, and to the heroic healthcare workers who are risking their lives to end this scourge.

Author's Acknowledgments

I want to express thanks to the team at John Wiley & Sons, Inc., for having asked me to participate in this important and exciting project. The core team that I have been working with to make this book come to life includes Sarah Sypniewski, contributor, Chad Sievers, project editor, and Tracy Boggier, senior acquisitions editor. You have helped keep me going at every step along the way. Sarah, it has been an honor and a pleasure to work with and to learn from you during the process of writing this book. In addition, I want to thank Kathy Nebenhaus at Wiley, without whose invitation I would not have had the opportunity to engage in this project.

Finally, a special thank you to my parents, Seymour and the late Laura Chapnick, for their lifelong support and encouragement of my education and personal and professional development.

Publisher's Acknowledgments

Acquisitions Editor: Tracy Boggier

Project Editor: Chad R. Sievers

Copy Editor: Chad R. Sievers

Contributor: Sarah Sypniewski

Art Coordinator: Alicia B. South

Project Coordinator: Patrick Redmond

Cover Photos: ©iStock.com/wildpixel